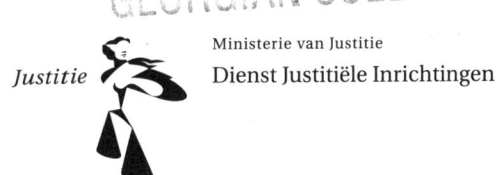

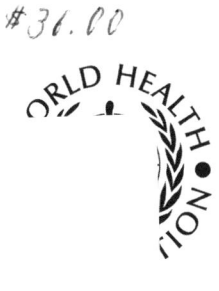

Ministerie van Justitie
Dienst Justitiële Inrichtingen

Health in prisons

A WHO guide to the essentials in prison health

Edited by: Lars Møller, Heino Stöver,
Ralf Jürgens, Alex Gatherer and Haik Nikogosian

Promoting health in prisons   The essentials

Abstract

Based on the experience of many countries in Europe and the advice of experts, this guide outlines some of the steps prison systems should take to reduce the public health risks from compulsory detention in often unhealthy situations, to care for prisoners in need and to promote the health of prisoners and staff. This especially requires that everyone working in prisons understand well how imprisonment affects health and the health needs of prisoners and that evidence-based prison health services can be provided for everyone needing treatment, care and prevention in prison. Other essential elements are being aware of and accepting internationally recommended standards for prison health; providing professional care with the same adherence to professional ethics as in other health services; and, while seeing individual needs as the central feature of the care provided, promoting a whole-prison approach to the care and promoting the health and well-being of those in custody.

Keywords

HEALTH PROMOTION – organization and administration
HEALTH SERVICES – standards
PRIMARY HEALTH CARE – standards
PRISONS
PRISONERS
QUALITY OF HEALTH CARE
HEALTH PLANNING GUIDELINES
EUROPE

EUR/07/5063925   ISBN 978 92 890 78209

Address requests about publications of the WHO Regional Office for Europe to:
    Publications
    WHO Regional Office for Europe
    Scherfigsvej 8
    DK-2100 Copenhagen Ø, Denmark
Alternatively, complete an online request form for documentation, health information, or for permission to quote or translate, on the Regional Office web site (http://www.euro.who.int/pubrequest).

© World Health Organization 2007
All rights reserved. The Regional Office for Europe of the World Health Organization welcomes requests for permission to reproduce or translate its publications, in part or in full.
The designations employed and the presentation of the material in this publication do not imply the expression of any opinion whatsoever on the part of the World Health Organization concerning the legal status of any country, territory, city or area or of its authorities, or concerning the delimitation of its frontiers or boundaries. Where the designation "country or area" appears in the headings of tables, it covers countries, territories, cities, or areas. Dotted lines on maps represent approximate border lines for which there may not yet be full agreement.
The mention of specific companies or of certain manufacturers' products does not imply that they are endorsed or recommended by the World Health Organization in preference to others of a similar nature that are not mentioned. Errors and omissions excepted, the names of proprietary products are distinguished by initial capital letters.
The World Health Organization does not warrant that the information contained in this publication is complete and correct and shall not be liable for any damages incurred as a result of its use. The views expressed by authors or editors do not necessarily represent the decisions or the stated policy of the World Health Organization.

Contents

Foreword vii
Preface viii
Contributors x
Definitions xvi

1. **Introduction** 1
   Who this guide is for 1
   How to use this guide 1
   The essentials and important first steps 1
   Political leadership 2
   Management leadership 3
   Leadership by each member of the staff 4
   The special leadership role of health personnel 4
   Partnerships for health: (1) the role of prisoners 5
   Partnerships for health: (2) community support 5
   References 5

2. **Standards in prison health: the prisoner as a patient** - *Andrew Coyle* 7
   The basic principles 7
   The relationship between the prisoner and health care staff 8
   The organization of prison health care 9
   European Prison Rules 11
   Conclusion 12
   References 12
   Further reading 13

3. **Protecting and promoting health in prisons: a settings approach** - *Paul Hayton* 15
   Introduction 15
   Major problems that need to be addressed 15
   The whole-prison or settings approach and a vision for a health-promoting prison 17
   References 20
   Further reading 20

4. **Primary health care in prisons** - *Andrew Fraser* 21
   Introduction 21
   The components of primary care 24
   The journey of primary care 24
   Prison health care resources 25
   Common problems encountered in primary care practice in prisons 26
   Building blocks for primary care in prison 26
   Measuring performance in health care 27
   Conclusion 30
   References 31
   Further reading 31

5. **Prison-specific ethical and clinical problems** - *Jean-Pierre Restellini* 33
   Introduction 33
   Health care staff in prison 34
   Disciplinary measures 35
   Physical restraint 36
   Intimate body searches 36

Prisoners who stop eating or go on hunger strikes 37
Torture and inhumane or degrading treatment 40
Conclusions 41
Reference 41
Further reading 41

6. **Communicable diseases -** *Dumitru Laticevschi* **43**
Introduction 43
Bloodborne diseases 45
Tuberculosis 47
Sexually transmitted infections 50
Skin conditions 56
Infectious diseases of the digestive tract 57
Reference 58
Further reading 59

7. **HIV infection and human rights in prisons -** *Rick Lines* **61**
Setting the context: HIV-related stigma and discrimination in prisons 61
Confidentiality in prison 62
HIV testing and pretest and post-test counselling 64
Coercive approaches are counterproductive 65
Addressing concerns about trust and confidentiality: working with nongovernmental organizations, people living with HIV, peers and professionals outside the prison system 68
Compassionate or early release 69
Conclusion 69
References 70
Further reading 70

8. **Tuberculosis control in prisons -** *Jaap Veen* **73**
Introduction 73
What is tuberculosis? 74
What can be done to reduce the risk of transmission of tuberculosis? 76
How to manage tuberculosis cases 79
Treatment 79
How should tuberculosis services in the penitentiary system be organized? 80
Conclusion 82
References 82
Further reading 83

9. **Drug use and drug services in prisons -** *Heino Stöver and Caren Weilandt* **85**
Drug use and the consequences for prisoners, prisons and prison health care 85
Definition of a drug user 87
Nature and prevalence of drug use and related risks in prisons 88
Prevention, treatment, harm reduction and aftercare 90
Organization and practice of health care, treatment and assistance 91
Assessment of drug problems and related infectious diseases 94
Preventing drug use 95
Detoxification 95
Drug-free units 97
Contract treatment units and drug-free units 97
Abstinence-oriented treatment and therapeutic communities in prison 98
Substitution treatment 99
Counselling and peer support 100
Harm reduction programmes 101
Involvement of community services 105
Vocational training 109
References 109
Further reading 111

10. **Substitution treatment in prisons -** *Andrej Kastelic* **113**
Introduction 113
What is substitution treatment? 114
The main goals of substitution treatment 115
Evidence of the benefits of substitution treatment 116
Effective treatment 120

Evidence of the benefits of substitution treatment 116
Effective treatment 120
Criteria for treatment and treatment plan 121
Risks and limitations 122
Substitution agents 122
Some basic information about treatment 126
The link with treatment for HIV infection 128
Special considerations for women 128
Future perspectives 129
References 129
Further reading 130

11. Mental health in prisons - *Eric Blaauw and Hjalmar J.C. van Marle* 133
Mental health and mental illness in prisons 133
Mental harm reduction and mental health promotion 134
Levels of care 135
Basic circumstances 137
Staff training 139
Conclusion 141
Mental health promotion in prisons: a checklist 141
References 144

12. Dental health in prisons - *Amit Bose and Tony Jenner* 147
Introduction 147
Dental health needs in prisons 148
Challenges in providing dental care to prisoners 148
Oral health promotion 149
Organization of prison dental services 150
Models of good practice 151
Conclusion 155
Further reading 155

13. Special health requirements for female prisoners - *Jan Palmer* 157
Introduction 157
Mental health problems 158
Suicidal behaviour in prisons 159
Substance use 161
Pregnancy 164
Children 165
Sexually transmitted infections 166
Bloodborne viruses 166
Violence 166
General health issues 167
References 169
Further reading 169

14. Promoting health and managing stress among prison employees - *Heiner Bögemann* 171
Introduction 171
Research on the health of prison employees 172
Risk factors and stress among prison employees 172
Frequent psychosocial risk factors in prisons 173
Promoting and developing employees with health in mind 174
Practical approaches to health promotion: best practices 174
Comprehensive health promotion for prison employees 175
Example of a health in prison project with important milestones 175
Essentials for active health management in prisons 176
Health promotion self-help networks in prisons 177
Continuing education 178
Results and prospects 178
References 179

Foreword

A continuing challenge in public health is to get services to the people who need them the most, especially those who are hardest to reach. Yet it is a sad reality of life that, at any one time, a high proportion of those with multiple health problems are incarcerated in the prisons of each country. They are certainly reachable, for a certain period at least.

For more than a decade, WHO has had a network of countries of the European region (with more than 30 countries now involved) supported by senior representatives approved at the ministerial level that gather to exchange experiences and evidence on how best to make prisons healthier places for staff as well as prisoners. The detection of serious communicable diseases such as HIV infection and tuberculosis, accompanied by adequate treatment and the introduction of harm reduction measures as necessary, contributes significantly to the health status of the communities from which the prisoners come and to which they return. In addition, it is now known that substance dependence can satisfactorily be treated in prisons. The many imprisoned people who have mental health problems can also be helped.

More recent developments include the real possibility that the time in custody can be used to promote healthier lifestyles, with better control over smoking and alcohol and perhaps over the use of violence in interpersonal relationships. An information database has been developed to obtain a measure of progress throughout the European region.

I commend this guide as a worthwhile way of reducing the risks to public health from inadequate services and as a way of promoting health and welfare among some highly disadvantaged people. This can contribute to reducing inequity in health.

It is increasingly being recognized that good prison health is good public health.

Dr Nata Menabde
Deputy Regional Director
WHO Regional Office for Europe

Preface

One of the strongest lessons from the end of the last century is that public health can no longer afford to ignore prison health. The rise and rapid spread of HIV infection and AIDS, the resurgence of other serious communicable diseases such as tuberculosis and hepatitis and the increasing recognition that prisons are inappropriate receptacles for people with dependence and mental health problems have thrust prison health high on the public health agenda. As all societies try to cope with these serious health problems, it has become clear that any national strategy for controlling them requires developing and including prison policies, as prisons contain, at any one time, a disproportionate number of those requiring health assistance.

Good prison health creates considerable benefits. It prevents the spread of diseases and promotes health through awareness of what everyone can do to help maintain their own health and well-being and that of others. In addition, however, it can help to improve the health status of communities, thus contributing to health for all.

This guide gives practical information and advice on how to achieve good health in prisons. Its advice is based on evidence of what works best, and the advice comes from selected experts with considerable knowledge of and experience in the special needs of prisons and places of compulsory detention. It outlines what is known now, but care will be taken to get regular feedback from those who wrote it and those who are using it, so that the guide can be updated regularly.

All prisons are different, but they share common challenges. Countries vary considerably in the resources available for improving prison services. The current position of prison health services varies substantially in prisons throughout the world. Some countries with basic or rudimentary services will need support to introduce the approaches indicated in this publication. Others are in more favourable positions. But we believe that all countries will find some areas of their prison health services that could be improved and will gain from careful consideration of this guide.

To address prison health in Europe in a multidisciplinary fashion, we approached 16 authors with expertise in both prison and public health and asked them to draft a chapter that covered the most important areas of prison health, the close connection with public health and looking ahead. We are very pleased that all the authors responded so effectively to our request.

The Editorial Board comprised:
- Jonathan Beynon, International Committee of the Red Cross, Switzerland;
- Alex Gatherer, Health in Prisons Project, WHO Regional Office for Europe;
- Paul Hayton, Prison Health, Department of Health, United Kingdom;
- Haik Nikogosian, Division of Health Programmes, WHO Regional Office for Europe;
- Eva Koprolin, Pompidou Group, Council of Europe, France;
- Marzena Ksel, Prison Health Services, Poland;
- Lucia Mihailescu, General Directorate of Penitentiaries, Romania;
- Lars Møller, Health in Prisons Project, WHO Regional Office for Europe;
- Edoardo Spacca, Cranstoun Drug Services, United Kingdom;
- Terhi Viljanen, European Institute for Crime Prevention and Control, Finland; and
- Caren Weilandt, Scientific Institute of the German Medical Association, Germany.

A special thanks to the Public Health Programme of the European Commission and to the Dutch Ministry of Health, Welfare and Sports for co-sponsoring this publication, to Ms Gerda van't Hoff, National Agency of Correctional Services, Ministry of Justice and to Nina Koch, Project Assistant, Health in Prisons Project,

WHO Regional Office for Europe.

Lars Møller, Heino Stöver, Ralf Jürgens, Alex Gatherer and Haik Nikogosian
Health in Prisons Project
WHO Regional Office for Europe

Contributors

Eric Blaauw

Eric Blaauw is treatment coordinator at Bouman GGZ Parole and senior researcher at the Department of (Forensic) Psychiatry of the University Erasmus Medical Centre in Rotterdam. He received his PhD on research on police custody procedures but has specialized on research on mental disorders, guidance programmes and suicide risk in penal institutions. His further interests include the psychology of stalking and the use of offender profiling for criminal investigations. Eric Blaauw has published more than 60 articles and book chapters and 8 books on these matters.

Heiner Bögemann

Heiner Bögemann has a Master of Public Health and PhD and is a social worker and psychosocial counsellor. He has been working for many years with people released from prisons, including more than 10 years as a probation officer. From 1997 to 2000 he headed a project focusing on health promotion and stress coping for prison staff. His practical experiences in health management in prisons became basis of the innovative foundation of the Health Centre for Prison Staff in Lower Saxony – the first and only centre of its kind in Germany. His position now is a coordinator of the network supporting health issues for more than 4000 staff members. Moreover, he is a member of the statewide crisis intervention team in prisons.

Amit Bose

Amit Bose is currently the Policy Manager for Oral Health and Dental Education for the United Kingdom Department of Health. Prior to his current appointment, he was District Performance Improvement Manager at the Department of Work and Pensions. He has also worked for Post Office Counters Ltd, where in 2000 he was part of the national team responsible for computerizing all the post office outlets in England.

Andrew Coyle

Andrew Coyle is Professor of Prison Studies at Kings College, University of London. Between 1997 and 2005 he was also Director of the International Centre for Prison Studies. Previous to that he worked for 25 years at a senior level in the prison services of the United Kingdom, during which time he governed four major prisons. He is a prison adviser to the United Nations High Commissioner for Human Rights, the United Nations Latin American Institute, the Council of Europe, including its Committee for the Prevention of Torture, and several national governments. He is a member of the United Kingdom Foreign Secretary's Expert Committee against Torture. He has a PhD in criminology from the University of Edinburgh. He is a

Fellow of King's College London and was appointed a Companion of the Order of St Michael and St George in 2003 for his contribution to international penal reform.

Andrew Fraser

Andrew Fraser is Director of Health and Care at the Scottish Prison Service, United Kingdom. He had worked as a public health specialist since 1993. Between 1997 and 2003, he was Deputy Chief Medical Officer with responsibility for public health policy at the Scottish Executive. From 1994 to 1997, he was Director of Public Health at National Health Service Highland. From 1993 to 1994, he was the Medical Director of the National Services Division, National Services Scotland. His main current interests are in prison health service reform, prison health as part of public health, national policy on alcohol problems, ethics and human rights. He is a member of the Steering Group of the WHO European Region Health and Prisons Project, a Member of the Council of the Royal College of Physicians of Edinburgh, the Board of the Faculty of Public Health in the United Kingdom and a Fellow of the Royal College of Physicians and Surgeons of Glasgow. He trained in medicine and public health in the Universities of Aberdeen and Glasgow and subsequently trained in internal medicine before embarking on a public health career.

Alex Gatherer

Alex Gatherer was director of public health for Oxford for many years and an Honorary Visiting Fellow of Green College, University of Oxford. He has been an adviser to the WHO European Health in Prisons Project since its inception and in 2006 was awarded the Alwyn Smith Prize of the Faculty of Public Health, Royal College of Physicians, London, partly in recognition of his work in public health and prisons.

Paul Hayton

Paul Hayton is Director of the Healthy Prisons Programme within the Healthy Settings Development Unit, School of Postgraduate Medicine, University of Central Lancashire, England. He is involved in research and development in prison health for the United Kingdom Department of Health and is Deputy Director of the WHO European Collaborating Centre for Health and Prisons, Department of Health. He has written several articles on prisons and health promotion and contributed to books on the subject. Prior to his current appointments, he held posts in the National Health Service concerned with public health development, specializing in HIV prevention. Previously he served in the Royal Air Force.

Tony Jenner

Tony Jenner is currently the Acting Deputy Chief Dental Officer at the Department of Health in England and has been Head of Oral Health Policy in the Department since 2003. He was appointed a Specialist in Dental Public Health in 1992 and also the Regional Dental Officer for the North West Region of England, United Kingdom. He has worked both in full-time National Health Service dental practice and the public dental service since 1971 prior to undertaking postgraduate research. He jointly led the development of the Department of Health and HM Prison Service's strategy for modernizing prison dental services in England, United Kingdom and has been the lead for prison dental health in the Department since 2002. He also led the development of the United Kingdom Government's Oral Health Strategy for England, United Kingdom, "Choosing Better Oral Health". He is a Fellow of the United Kingdom Faculty of Public Health and the Faculty of General Dental Practice United Kingdom.

Ralf Jürgens
Ralf Jürgens is a co-founder of the Canadian HIV/AIDS Legal Network and was its Executive Director from 1998 to November 2004. Since December 2004, he has worked as a consultant on HIV and AIDS, health, policy and human rights in Burkina Faso, Canada, Kenya, the Russian Federation, Senegal, Tajikistan, Ukraine and Zambia for organizations such as the International HIV/AIDS Alliance, the Open Society Institute, WHO, the United Nations Office on Drugs and Crime, the International Affairs Directorate of Health Canada and the Canadian HIV/AIDS Legal Network. Previously, he was Project Coordinator of the Canadian Expert Committee on AIDS and Prisons and taught the first course on AIDS and the law ever to be offered at a university in Canada. He is a member of the Join United Nations Programme on HIV/AIDS (UNAIDS) Global Reference Group on HIV/AIDS and Human Rights and recently co-chaired the Policy Track of the XVI International AIDS Conference in 2006. Ralf Jürgens is the author of many reports and more than 100 articles on legal, ethical and human rights issues related to HIV and AIDS and has edited a number of journals on HIV and AIDS and on prison issues. He has a Master's Degree in Law from McGill University, Montreal, Canada, and a doctorate in law from the University of Munich, Germany.

Andrej Kastelic
Andrej Kastelic is a physician and head of the National Centre for Treatment of Drug Addiction in Ljubljana, Slovenia. Further, he is the head of the Coordination of the Centres for the Prevention and Treatment of Drug Addiction at the Ministry of Health of the Republic of Slovenia and President of the Board of Directors. Andrej Kastelic is the President of the South-eastern Europe Adriatic Addiction Treatment Network, the Director of the Board of the Sound of Reflection Foundation, consultant for treatment programmes in prisons at the Ministry of Justice of Slovenia and consultant and/or principal trainer in developing drug dependence treatment programmes in communities and prisons in Albania, Azerbaijan, Bosnia and Herzegovina, Montenegro, Romania, Republic of Serbia, Taiwan, The former Yugoslav Republic of Macedonia, and Ukraine. He serves as a technical adviser to the International Harm Reduction Development Program and is a member of the provisional substitution treatment working groups at WHO, UNAIDS and the United Nations Office on Drugs and Crime, consultant for the Organization for Security and Co-operation in Europe, UNAIDS and member of Expert Committee that has prepared and reviewed European Union methadone guidelines. Andrej Kastelic has written more than 300 books and articles on drug dependence and several manuals and leaflets for drug users and on preventing drug use.

Dumitru Laticevschi
Dumitru Laticevschi is a physician and worked as a surgeon at the Central Penitentiary Hospital in the Republic of Moldova since 1995. From 1997 to 1999 he was involved in designing, from 2000 to 2003 in managing and from 2003 to 2006 in advising the prison tuberculosis programme for the Republic of Moldova. In 2000

he designed and implemented the pilot project on needle and syringe exchange in prisons of the Republic of Moldova. From 2003 to 2006 he managed the Republic of Moldova's Tuberculosis (TB)/AIDS Programme Implementation Unit, financed by the World Bank and the Global Fund to Fight AIDS, Tuberculosis and Malaria. Since April 2006, Dumitru Laticevschi has been working at the Global Fund, as the Fund Portfolio Manager for tuberculosis, HIV and malaria grants for several eastern European countries.

Rick Lines

Rick Lines, MA, LLM, is the Executive Director of the Irish Penal Reform Trust, Ireland's leading nongovernmental organization campaigning for prisoners' rights and prison reform. He has been working in prisoners' rights advocacy and policy reform since 1993 with nongovernmental organizations in Canada and Europe and is recognized internationally as an expert on HIV and AIDS, harm reduction, and drug policy in prisons. Rick Lines has been a member of several HIV and AIDS advisory committees of the Correctional Service of Canada and has served as a Technical Assistance Adviser to Romania's and Bulgaria's Ministries of Justice on behalf of United Nations agencies. He is coauthor of HIV/AIDS prevention, care, treatment and support in prison settings: a framework for an effective national response, published jointly by the United Nations, WHO and UNAIDS in 2006. He is a member of the Editorial Board of the International Journal of Prisoner Health. Rick Lines has spoken internationally before many audiences, and his articles have appeared in HIV/AIDS Policy & Law Review, the European Human Rights Law Review and the International Journal of Prisoner Health.

Lars Møller

Lars Møller is a physician with a specialization in public health medicine and in 1998 obtained a doctoral degree in medicine from the University of Copenhagen, Denmark. He worked at the Institute of Public Health, University of Copenhagen in the field of epidemiology and disease prevention and for the National Board of Health in Copenhagen. From 1992 to 2001, he worked as a medical consultant for the International Rehabilitation Council for Torture Victims. He has been working for the WHO Regional Office for Europe since 2001 and has managed the WHO European Health in Prisons Project since 2002.

Haik Nikogosian

Dr Haik Nikogosian is currently with the WHO Regional Office for Europe, serving as Deputy Director, Division of Health Programmes, and Unit Head, Noncommunicable Diseases and Mental Health. He holds an MD, PhD and Doctor of Science in health care and public health, and has been Professor of Medical Sciences since 1993. Previously Chairman of the Armenian Diagnostic Services Centre, Chairman of the National Institute of Health of Armenia, and visiting professor in the University of Maryland, USA, he later served as the Minister of Health of Armenia before joining WHO Regional Office for Europe in 2000. Coordinating the work on alcohol, drugs and health in prisons has been one of the important areas of his work at WHO over the recent years.

Jan Palmer

Jan Palmer is a Nurse Consultant in Substance Misuse and has led the development of clinical substance misuse services in women's prisons for the past 10 years. During that time she wrote and implemented a set of clinical guidelines that were the first national prison protocols in western Europe. Based within prison health at the Department of Health, Jan is now also offering support and advice to some of the adult male prison estate as they also seek to develop their clinical substance misuse services. Jan Palmer's particular areas of professional interest include the care of pregnant drug users and the reduction of self-harm and self-inflicted deaths in custody. Prior to beginning this work in prisons, Jan Palmer worked in a community substance misuse service, which was preceded by 17 years working in adult mental health services, including the care of those with a dual diagnosis.

Jean-Pierre Restellini
Jean-Pierre Restellini, MD, LLB is a designated Member of the Committee for the Prevention of Torture at the Council of Europe on behalf of Switzerland. He is a Management Member of the Swiss Training Centre for Penitentiary Personnel and former Member of the Central Ethics Commission of the Swiss Academy of Medical Sciences.

Heino Stöver
Heino Stöver is a social scientist and Professor of Public Health at the Department of Education at the Carl von Ossietzky University of Oldenburg, Germany. Since 1987 he has been Director of the Archive and Documentation Centre for Drug Literature and Research at the University of Bremen (www.archido.de). He is cofounder of the Bremen Institute for Drug Research (BISDRO) and Senior Expert of the Gesellschaft für technische Zusammenarbeit (GTZ) in Berlin, Germany. Heino Stöver's main fields of expertise are health provision, drug services, prisons and related health issues. His research and consultancy expertise include working as a consultant for the European Commission, United Nations Office on Drugs and Crime, WHO, European Monitoring Centre for Drugs and Drug Addiction, International Committee of the Red Cross and Open Society Institute in various contexts. Currently, Heino Stöver is carrying out research for a major project on problematic drug and alcohol users in police detention funded by the European Union framework programme on police and judicial cooperation on criminal matters (AGIS), two other research projects in the AGIS line funded by the European Union and a European study on harm reduction in European prisons (European Network on Drugs and Infections Prevention in Prison research). He has published several articles and books on substitution programmes (including the provision of heroin) in the community and in prisons, health issues in prisons and is the joint editor of the *International Journal of Prisoner Health*. Heino Stöver has gained project experience by participating in several projects in the European Union and is currently project leader in the twinning light project on capacity-building for institutions involved in surveillance and prevention of communicable diseases in the penitentiary system in Latvia.

Hjalmar J.C. van Marle
Hjalmar J.C. van Marle is Professor of Forensic Psychiatry at the Faculty of Medicine and the Faculty of Law of the Erasmus University Rotterdam. Further, he is working as a forensic psychiatrist and psychotherapist at the forensic outpatient clinic De Dok in Rotterdam and has a permanent appointment as an expert witness at

the Courts of Justice. He is also Chair of the Research Programme of the Expertise Centre for Forensic Psychiatry in Utrecht. Formerly he was chief of staff and medical superintendent, respectively, of the maximum-security hospital Dr S. van Mesdagkliniek in Groningen and of the forensic observation centre the Pieter Baan Centrum in Utrecht. For several years he was appointed as a psychiatric adviser at the Ministry of Justice as well as at the Prof. W.P.J. Pompekliniek in Nijmegen. He has been Professor of Forensic Psychiatry at the University of Nijmegen and psychotherapist at the Dr H. van der Hoeven TBS Hospital in Utrecht. He is former chair of the International Academy of Law and Mental Health and member of the editorial board of Forensische Psychiatrie und Psychologie, the *International Journal of Forensic Health* and Psychiatrienet.nl. Since 1979, Hjalmar J.C. van Marle has published on the diagnosis and treatment in custody of mentally disordered (sexual) delinquents, on dealing with aggression during treatment, on the research of recidivism and the mental risk factors and on national as well as international policy in forensic psychiatry. Current fields of research are mental determinants of violent behaviour, persistent delinquency in adolescents, treatment effects and the epidemiology of criminality in combination with mental health care.

Jaap Veen
Jaap Veen, MD, PhD started his career as a Medical Officer in Botswana, where among other general duties he helped formulate the national tuberculosis programme of Botswana in 1976. From 1979 to 1989, he worked as a district dispensary tuberculosis specialist in the Netherlands. In 1980 he got a degree in public health and in 1992 his PhD. From 1989 to 2005 he worked as a tuberculosis consultant for the Royal Netherlands Tuberculosis Foundation (KNCV). Having been trained by Karel Styblo, from 1986 he was a tuberculosis consultant for various agencies, including WHO and the World Bank, in countries in Africa and Asia and since 1996 in eastern Europe. For KNCV he coordinated the Tuberculosis in Prison Projects in Kazakhstan and the Republic of Moldova and was a consultant for the International Committee of the Red Cross Tuberculosis Control in Prison projects in the southern Caucasus. Since 2005 he has been the Tuberculosis Regional Medical Director of Project HOPE in Central Asia. In 2005 he was awarded an Honorary Doctorate in the Republic of Moldova.

Caren Weilandt
Caren Weilandt is a psychologist and psychotherapist specializing in psychophysiology, clinical psychology and health promotion. She has a PhD in psychology from the Free University of Berlin. She has worked at the Scientific Institute of the German Medical Association (WIAD, Bonn, Germany) since 1988 and is the deputy managing director of the Institute. She was involved in several studies on HIV prevention on behalf of Germany's Federal Ministry of Health and the European Commission. Her research activities comprise studies on psychoneuroimmunology and HIV infection, migration and health, infectious diseases and drug use. She has developed educational programmes on HIV prevention for several professional groups. Since 1996 she has coordinated the European Network on HIV/AIDS Prevention in Prisons and is currently coordinating the European Network on Drugs and Infections Prevention in Prison funded by the European Commission.

Definitions

The term **prison** is intended to denote, as a minimum, the institutions that hold people who have been sentenced to a period of imprisonment by the courts for offences against the law. However, the principles, approaches and technical advice in this guide are relevant to other forms of compulsory detention. The institutions included in the term prison can vary between countries.

The phrase health promoting prison is used to cover the prisons in which: the risks to health are reduced to a minimum; essential prison duties such as the maintenance of security are undertaken in a caring atmosphere that recognizes the inherent dignity of every prisoner and their human rights; health services are provided to the level and in a professional manner equivalent to what is provided in the country as a whole; and a whole-prison approach to promoting health and welfare is the norm.

1. Introduction

Who this guide is for
This guide has been created for everyone who works in a prison or has a part to play in promoting the health of prisoners and/or staff. Although this naturally includes health care professionals, this guide will provide useful information and guidance to all individuals and organizations responsible for prisoners and, in addition, will assist everyone who has anything to do with prisons.

Everyone has a part to play to make prisons healthier places for both staff and inmates and to ensure that health protection and health promotion activities in prison can be successful. Applying the recommendations in this guide will produce a prison with satisfying roles for staff members and a marked reduction in the harm that imprisonment can create.

How to use this guide
Each chapter takes a similar approach. It starts with a list of key facts and issues and then provides background information and considers the problem and what can be done in detail.
The guide takes a whole-prison approach. We therefore suggest that everyone read the definitions, preface and the first three chapters, and only then should they concentrate on the particular area of their work or interest to be able to assess current practice and change it if required.

The essentials and important first steps
Although individuals committed to particular parts of the prison service can do much, we strongly believe that a health promoting prison can only be achieved if all staff are involved, including senior staff members who determine the ethos of the prison as a whole.

Changes should be introduced with continuity in mind. Although single-issue and often externally funded initiatives and pilot projects can achieve much, projects will be more effective in the longer term if the prison health system is based on the characteristics of a sustainable approach, that is with sound policies based on explicit principles that lead to effective practices by well-supported and trained staff.

Sustainability can best be achieved if strong links are created between prison health care services and the health services of the local community and if they work in close cooperation. Such collaboration will help to prevent prisons from being used as default health care services.

Many essential components are required to achieve a health promoting prison, including political leadership, management leadership and leadership by each staff member. Health care staff members have a special role to play, but prisoners also have a role, and community support is important.

Political leadership

The important first steps start with political leadership (Box 1.1).

Box 1.1. Important first steps for achieving a healthy prison
1. political leadership
   1.1 recognize that prisons perform a vital public service
   1.2 understand how good prison health affects public health
   1.3 support close collaboration between prison health and national health services
   1.4 support intercountry learning: for example, check whether your country is a member of the WHO Health in Prisons Project;
2. establish national policy through advice from senior staff members in the prison services and senior health policy advisers; and
3. check that prison staff members have easy access to key documents, such as this guide, in their own language or another language they understand.

It is not sufficiently recognized that the prison service is a public service, meeting some fundamental needs of society, such as the need to feel safe and to feel that crime is sufficiently punished and reparations made. As with all public services, the extent and the quality of provision depend on a political decision. Political support for healthier prisons should be based on the recognition that:
- good prison health is essential to good public health;
- good public health will make good use of the opportunities presented by prisons; and
- prisons can contribute to the health of communities by helping to improve the health of some of the most disadvantaged people in society.

Experience in several countries of Europe has drawn attention to the problems that often arise if prison health services are provided separately from the country's public health services. These include difficulty in recruiting professional staff and inadequate continuing education and training. It is now strongly recommended that prison health services work closely with national health services and health ministries, so that the prisons can provide the same standard of care as local hospitals and communities. Indeed, as the WHO Moscow Declaration on Prison Health as a Part of Public Health (WHO Regional Office for Europe, 2003) acknowledged, the government ministry responsible for prison health should, where possible, be the ministry responsible for public health services.

Because prison services throughout Europe face similar public health issues and can learn a lot from each other, most of the Member States have come together and participate in the WHO Health in Prisons Project. In countries that are not currently members of the Project, it is suggested that the health ministry raise with WHO the question of either membership or association, so that these countries could also benefit from the Project and hear of developments and experiences that may be relevant to them.

The need to change and improve practices can best be accepted, and change achieved, if the people concerned have the knowledge, appropriate attitudes and the understanding as to why their practice should be different. This guide should help countries that seek reform in meeting these needs, but the guide will have to be available in a language the staff can understand. The most important immediate step for policy-makers to take may be to ensure that this guide is translated for their prison staff.

Management leadership

Prisons in modern societies are complex places to manage. The phenomenon of prison overcrowding, the epidemics of serious life-threatening diseases, the continued use of prisons for housing mentally ill people and the high levels of substance abuse in many countries have all contributed to increasing the pressures on management at all levels.

Box 1.2. Important areas for prison managers to monitor
1. reception, aiming to reduce stress;
2. induction, to enhance coping skills;
3. general environment, for cleanliness;
4. general environment, to be "controlled", with staff in charge of the whole prison at all times;
5. support for prisoners, mentor or key worker schemes;
6. support and recognition for staff;
7. contact with families, friends and the outside community;
8. basic life skills such as reading, writing and arithmetic;
9. activities available, including work, educational, active leisure;
10. privacy and maintaining confidentiality; and
11. individuality, providing choice where possible.

Most prisoners nowadays have multiple problems. Add in the detention of asylum-seekers and the high levels of imprisonment among people from ethnic minorities, and this all produces a very challenging environment for those required to guarantee security, safety and decency. We hope that this guide will be of value in showing how many of the above-mentioned problems can best be addressed.

Managers, leading from the top but also well supported by ministerial or national staff, have the first challenge: determining the ethos, the overall feel of the prison. A management checklist in a publication of the WHO Health in Prisons Project dealing with mental health promotion in prisons (WHO Regional Office for Europe, 1999) starts with the sentence: "A concept of care, positive expectations and respect should permeate all prisons."

The checklist then considers other important areas for managers to monitor (Box 1.2). Some prison managers have found including senior health staff in their top management group to be useful, so that all aspects of prison life can be assessed in terms of their contribution to health. Where the public health service employs health personnel, their regular involvement in prison management helps to reduce the difficulties that can arise when those responsible for the control and safety regime work alongside a health staff with its own, different, professional codes. Some tension between health and security staff may be inevitable, but this can be reduced considerably if different staff understand and learn to respect each other's roles.

Leadership by each member of the staff
A health promoting prison cannot be created without the contribution of each member of its staff. Given the current health problems in prisons, staff members need to know and understand what the health problems are, how infections can spread, how they can be better controlled and how health and well-being can be promoted.

If a duty of care, explicitly or implicitly, is imposed on staff in prisons, they must have the knowledge and the understanding of what this means for their everyday practices. A guide such as this should help considerably to provide the knowledge that is necessary, but staff should have opportunities to develop further the understanding that is so important for issues relating to health, including ethical ones.

Health promoting prisons do not focus solely on prisoner health. The health and well-being of staff is equally important. Working in prison often involves being confronted with difficult health matters, violence, bullying, mobbing and mental health problems as well as with poor quality and overcrowded living conditions for prisoners, with severe consequences on their psychosocial well-being.

Many prisons experience an increasing absence rate due to illness among staff members. This indicates how prisons affect the health of everyone working there, along with other phenomena such as burnout, alcohol and drug abuse, internal withdrawal and the inability to cope with traumatic experiences in daily work. The health status of staff should therefore be reviewed regularly, with top management paying attention to such indicators as staff sickness and staff turnover levels.

Box 1.3 provides a checklist of initiatives that can help in maintaining the health of staff, increase their information and understanding and help them promote their own health and well-being.

Box 1.3. Checklist of health initiatives of and for staff in prisons
1. setting up health promotion groups;
2. introducing information and health days focusing on drug use, alcohol, nutrition, infectious diseases, violence and gender-specific issues;
3. conducting non-smoking training;
4. improving nutrition during working hours, such as fruit during canteen meals;
5. ensuring that colleagues can consult on problems and crises;
6. setting up regional working groups for exchanging experience; and
7. setting up help structures after special incidents and stress-related illness (contact with colleagues and debriefing).

The special leadership role of health personnel
Physicians and nurses and other professionals working in prisons have a unique leadership role in producing the health promoting prison. They should start from a sound basis of professional training in which issues such as confidentiality, patient rights and human rights have been fully covered and discussed. They should also have some knowledge of epidemiology, of how diseases spread and of how lifestyles and socioeconomic background factors can influence ill health. They should also be aware of human nutrition and of the importance of exercise and fresh air in pro-

moting health. They should be alert to potential threats to health and able to detect early signs of mental health problems.

All staff should be aware of what health staff can do and can be asked to do but also of the activities in which health staff should never be involved.

Partnerships for health: (1) the role of prisoners
One of the central pillars of health promotion is the concept of empowerment: the individual has to be able to make healthy choices and has to be allowed to do so. In health promotion in prisons, this approach is not possible. It is therefore important that as much empowerment as possible be built into the prison regime.

One area that has been found to be important is providing health information to prisoners. Fact sheets should be made available for prisoners suffering from chronic ailments such as diabetes, explaining what the prison health service can provide and providing advice as to how the prisoner can best cope with such an illness while in prison. If written fact sheets will not be effective, because of language barriers or poor literacy, alternative ways of sharing information should be used, such as the use of videos and other visual aids or health discussion groups with a trained health worker.

Selected fact and advisory sheets can be produced based on this guide and adapted for use where necessary.

Partnerships for health: (2) community support
Regular contact with local community services and the involvement of voluntary agencies can assist greatly in promoting health and well-being in prisons. Where possible, prisoners should be connected to key community services before leaving prison, such as probation or parole and social services.

References
United Nations (1966). *International Covenant on Economic, Social and Cultural Rights*. Geneva, Office of the United Nations High Commissioner for Human Rights (http://www.ohchr.org/english/law/cescr.htm, accessed 15 September 2006).
WHO Regional Office for Europe (2003). *Declaration on Prison Health as a Part of Public Health*. Copenhagen, WHO Regional Office for Europe 2003 (http://www.euro.who.int/Document/HIPP/moscow_declaration_eng04.pdf, accessed 15 September 2006).

2. Standards in prison health: the prisoner as a patient -

Andrew Coyle

Key points
- People who are in prison have the same right to health care as everyone else.
- Prison administrations have a responsibility to ensure that prisoners receive proper health care and that prison conditions promote the well-being of both prisoners and prison staff.
- Health care staff must deal with prisoners primarily as patients and not prisoners.
- Health care staff must have the same professional independence as their professional colleagues who work in the community.
- Health policy in prisons should be integrated into national health policy, and the administration of public health should be closely linked to the health services administered in prisons.
- This applies to all health matters but is particularly important for communicable diseases.
- The European Prison Rules of the Council of Europe provide important standards for prison health care.

The basic principles

Several international standards define the quality of health care that should be provided to prisoners. In the first place, the provision in Article 12 of the International Covenant on Economic, Social and Cultural Rights (United Nations, 1966) establishes "the right of everyone to the enjoyment of the highest attainable standard of physical and mental health". This applies to prisoners just as it does to every other human being. Those who are imprisoned retain their fundamental right to enjoy good health, both physical and mental, and retain their entitlement to a standard of health care that is at least the equivalent of that provided in the wider community.

The United Nations (1990) Basic Principles for the Treatment of Prisoners indicate how the entitlement of prisoners to the highest attainable standard of health care should be delivered: "Prisoners shall have access to the health services available in the country without discrimination on the grounds of their legal situation" (Principle 9). In other words, the fact that people are in prison does not mean that they have any reduced right to appropriate health care. Rather, the opposite is the case. When a state deprives people of their liberty, it takes on a responsibility to look after their health in terms both of the conditions under which it detains them and of the individual treatment that may be necessary. Prison administrations have a responsibility not simply to provide health care but also to establish conditions that promote the well-being of both prisoners and prison staff. Prisoners should not leave prison in a worse condition than when they entered. This principle is reinforced by Recommendation No. R (98) 7 of the Committee of Ministers of the Council of Europe (1998) concerning the ethical and organizational aspects of health care in prison and by the European Committee for the Prevention of Torture and Inhuman or Degrading Treatment or Punishment (CPT), particularly in its *3rd general report* (Council of Europe, 1993). The European Court of Human Rights is also producing an increasing body of case law confirming the obligation of states to safeguard the health of prisoners in their care.[1]

The argument is sometimes advanced that states cannot provide adequate health care for prisoners because of shortage of resources. In the 11th general report on its activities (Council of Europe, 2001), the CPT underlined the obligations state governments have to prisoners even in times of economic difficulty:

The CPT is aware that in periods of economic difficulties … sacrifices have to be made, including in penitentiary establishments. However, regardless of the difficulties faced at any given time, the act of depriving a person of his liberty always entails a duty of care which calls for effective methods of prevention, screening, and treatment. Compliance with this duty by public authorities is all the more important when it is a question of care required to treat life-threatening diseases.

In respect of the obligation to provide adequate health care to prisoners, there are two fundamental considerations. One concerns the relationship between the prisoner and the health care staff and the other concerns how prison health care is organized.

The relationship between the prisoner and health care staff

All health care staff members who work in prisons must always remember that their first duty to any prisoner who is their patient is clinical. This is underlined in the first of the United Nations (1982) Principles of Medical Ethics relevant to the Role of Health Personnel, particularly Physicians, in the Protection of Prisoners and Detainees against Torture and Other Cruel, Inhuman or Degrading Treatment or Punishment, which states:

Health personnel, particularly physicians, charged with the medical care of prisoners and detainees have a duty to provide them with protection of their physical and mental health and treatment of disease of the same quality and standard as is afforded to those who are not imprisoned or detained.

The International Council of Prison Medical Services confirmed this principle when it agreed on the Oath of Athens (Prison Health Care Practitioners, 1979):

We, the health professionals who are working in prison settings, meeting in Athens on September 10, 1979, hereby pledge, in keeping with the spirit of the Oath of Hippocrates, that we shall endeavour to provide the best possible health care for those who are incarcerated in prisons for whatever reasons, without prejudice and within our respective professional ethics.

This principle is particularly important for physicians. In some countries, full-time physicians can spend their whole career working in the prison environment. It is virtually inevitable in such situations that these physicians will form a close relationship with prison management and indeed may be members of the senior management team of the prison. One consequence of this may be that the director of the prison will occasionally expect the physician to assist in managing prisoners

---

[1] See, for example, the cases of *Mouisel v. France* (application number 67263/010), *Henaf v. France* (application number 65436/01) and *McGlinchey and others v. The United Kingdom* (application number 50390/99).

who are causing difficulty. For example, the security staff may ask the physician to sedate prisoners who are violent to themselves, to other prisoners or to staff. In some jurisdictions, prison administrations may demand that physicians provide them with confidential information about a person's HIV status. Physicians should never lose sight of the fact that their relationship with every prisoner should be first and foremost that between physician and patient. A physician should never do anything to patients or cause anything to be done to them that is not in their best clinical interests. Similarly, as with all other patients, physicians should always seek consent from the patient before taking any clinical action, unless the patient is not competent on clinical grounds to give this consent. An Internet diploma course entitled Doctors working in prison: human rights and ethical dilemmas provided free of charge on the Internet by the Norwegian Medical Association (2004) on behalf of the World Medical Association focuses on many of these issues.[2]

This primary duty to deal with prisoners as patients applies equally to other health care staff. In many countries nurses carry out many basic health care functions. These may include carrying out preliminary health assessments of newly admitted prisoners, issuing medicines or applying treatments prescribed by a physician or being the first point of contact for prisoners concerned about their health. The nurses who carry out these duties should be properly qualified for what they do and should treat people primarily as patients rather than as prisoners when carrying out their duties. The International Council of Nurses (1998) published a statement saying, among other things, that national nursing associations should provide access to confidential advice, counselling and support for prison nurses.

The organization of prison health care
One method of ensuring that prisoners have access to an appropriate quality of health care is by providing close links between prison-administered health services and public health. In recent years, some countries have begun to create and strengthen such relationships. However, many prison and public health reformers argue that a close relationship is not enough and that prison health should be part of the general health services of the country rather than a specialist service under the government ministry responsible for the prisons. There are strong arguments for moving in this direction in terms of improving the quality of health care provided to prisoners. In Norway, for example, the process of giving local health authorities responsibility for providing health care services in prison was completed in the 1980s. In France, legislation was introduced in 1994 placing prison health under the General Health Directorate for public health issues in the Ministry of Health. In England and Wales, United Kingdom, responsibility and also the budget for prison health care was transferred to the National Health Service in 2002.

The Committee of Ministers of the Council of Europe (1998) has urged that "health policy in custody should be integrated into, and compatible with, national health policy". The Committee points out that, as well as being in the interest of prisoners, this integration is in the interest of the health of the population at large, especially for policies relating to infectious diseases that can spread from prisons to the wider community. The vast majority of prisoners will return to civil society one day, often to the communities from which they have come. Some are in prison for very

[2] *World Medical Association Declaration on Hunger Strikers Adopted by the 43rd World Medical Assembly Malta, November 1991 and revised by the WMA General Assembly, Pilanesberg, South Africa, October 2006*

short periods. When they are released, it is important for the good of society that they return to society in good health rather than needing more support from the public health services or bringing infectious diseases with them. Continuity of care between prisons and communities is a public health imperative. Many other people go into and come out of prison on a daily basis: staff, lawyers, officials and other visitors. This means that there is significant potential for transmitting serious disease or infection. For these reasons, prisons cannot be seen as separate health sites from other institutions in society.

WHO strongly recommends that prison and public health care be closely linked. The Moscow Declaration on Prison Health as a Part of Public Health (WHO Regional Office for Europe, 2003) elaborated on some of the reasons why close working relationships with public health authorities are so important.
- Penitentiary populations contain an overrepresentation of members of the most marginalized groups in society, people with poor health and chronic untreated conditions, drug users, vulnerable people and those who engage in risky activities such as injecting drugs and commercial sex work.
- The movement of people already infected with or at high risk of disease to penitentiary institutions and back into civil society without effective treatment and follow-up gives rise to the risk of the spread of communicable diseases both within and beyond the penitentiary system. Prevention and treatment responses must be based on scientific evidence and on sound public health principles, with the involvement of the private sector, nongovernmental organizations and the affected population.
- The living conditions in most prisons of the world are unhealthy. Overcrowding, violence, lack of light, fresh air and clean water, poor food and infection-spreading activities such as tattooing are common. Rates of infection with tuberculosis, HIV and hepatitis are much higher than in the general population.

The Declaration makes a series of recommendations that would form the basis for improving the health care of all detained people, protecting the health of penitentiary personnel and contributing to the public health goals of every Member State in the European Region of WHO.
- Member States are recommended to develop close working links between the health ministry and the ministry responsible for the penitentiary system to ensure high standards of treatment for detainees, protection for personnel, joint training of professionals in modern standards of disease control, high levels of professionalism among penitentiary health care personnel, continuity of treatment between the penitentiary and outside society and unification of statistics.
- Member States are recommended to ensure that all necessary health care is provided to people deprived of their liberty free of charge.
- Public and penitentiary health systems are recommended to work together to ensure that harm reduction becomes the guiding principle of policy on preventing the transmission of HIV and hepatitis in penitentiary systems.
- Public and penitentiary health systems are recommended to work together to ensure that tuberculosis is detected early and is promptly and adequately treated and that transmission is prevented in penitentiary systems.

- State authorities, civil and penitentiary medical services, international organizations and the mass media are recommended to consolidate their efforts to develop and implement a complex approach to tackling the dual infection of tuberculosis and HIV.
- Governmental organizations, civil and penitentiary medical services and international organizations are recommended to promote their activities and consolidate their efforts to improve the quality of the psychological and psychiatric treatment provided to people who are imprisoned.
- Member States are recommended to work to improve prison conditions so that the minimum health requirements for light, air, space and nutrition are met.
- The WHO Regional Office for Europe is recommended to ensure that all its specialist departments and country officers take account in their work of the health care needs and problems of penitentiary systems and develop and coordinate activities to improve the health of detainees.

European Prison Rules
All the countries that are members of the WHO Health in Prisons Project are also members of the Council of Europe. The Committee of Ministers of the Council of Europe (1973) adopted the European Standard Minimum Rules for the Treatment of Prisoners, which were closely modelled on the Standard Minimum Rules for the Treatment of Prisoners adopted by the United Nations (Office of the United Nations High Commissioner for Human Rights, 1957). In 1973, the Council of Europe had 15 members. By the beginning of 1987, the Council had expanded to 21 members, and the Committee of Ministers of the Council of Europe (1987) had adopted a new set of European Prison Rules. At the time, the Committee of Ministers noted "that significant social trends and changes in regard to prison treatment and management have made it desirable to reformulate the Standard Minimum Rules for the Treatment of Prisoners, drawn up by the Council of Europe (Resolution (73) 5) so as to support and encourage the best of these developments and offer scope for future progress". The membership of the Council of Europe has expanded further to 46 states in 2005. For that reason, the Council of Europe decided to revise the 1987 European Prison Rules.

The revised European Prison Rules, adopted on 11 January 2006 by the Committee of Ministers of the Council of Europe (2006), contain a significantly expanded section on health care in the prison setting. For the first time, the European Prison Rules specifically refer to the obligation of prison authorities to safeguard the health of all prisoners (§39) and the need for prison medical services to be organized in close relationship with the general public health administration (§40).

Every prison is recommended to have the services of at least one qualified general medical practitioner and to have other personnel suitably trained in health care (§41). Arrangements to safeguard health care begin at the point of first admission, when prisoners are entitled to have a medical examination (§42), and continue throughout the course of detention (§43). The commentary to the European Prison Rules refers to some recent developments in imprisonment with implications for health care. One is the increasing tendency for courts to impose very long sentences, which increases the possibility that old prisoners may die in prison. Related to this is the need to give proper and humane treatment to any prisoner who is terminally ill. The Council of Europe (1998) has also made a recommendation on the treatment of prisoners who are on hunger strike. In addition to dealing with the health needs of individual prisoners, those responsible for prison health are also recommended to inspect the general conditions of detention, including food, water, hygiene, sanitation, heating, lighting and ventilation, as well as the suitability and cleanliness of the prisoners' clothing and bedding (§44). The European Prison Rules also recommend make provision for prisoners who require specialist treatment (§46) and those who have mental health needs (§47).

One important change should be noted. The 1987 European Prison Rules provided that prison authorities could only impose "punishment by disciplinary confinement and any other punishment which might have an adverse effect on the physical or mental health of the prisoner" provided that the medical officer certified in writing that the prisoner was fit to undergo such punishment. This led to concerns that, by providing this certification, the physician was in effect authorizing the imposition of punishment, in contradiction to the Hippocratic oath. The revised European Prison Rules remove this requirement.

Conclusion
This chapter has laid out the guiding principles for prison health care. The starting point is the principle that health care decisions must be made on clinical grounds and with the patient's interests and consent underlying every clinical judgement and action. Professional independence and patient autonomy, even within prisons, are crucial, as is the need for equivalence of care. It has been suggested that these requirements are most likely to be met if the arrangements for delivering health care in prison are closely linked to the provision of health care in the rest of society. These principles are linked to international human rights standards, including the revised European Prison Rules.

References
Committee of Ministers of the Council of Europe (1973). Resolution (73) 5, *The European Standard Minimum Rules for the Treatment of Prisoners (adopted by the Committee of Ministers on 19 January 1973)*. Strasbourg, Council of Europe, 1973.
Committee of Ministers of the Council of Europe (1987). *Recommendation No. R (87) 3 of the Committee of Ministers to Member States on the European Prison Rules (adopted by the Committee of Ministers on 12 February 1987)*. Strasbourg, Council of Europe.
Committee of Ministers of the Council of Europe (1998). *Recommendation No. R (98) 7 of the Committee of Ministers to Member States concerning the ethical and organisational aspects of health care in prison (adopted by the Committee of Ministers on 8 April 1998)*. Strasbourg, Council of Europe, 1998.
Committee of Ministers of the Council of Europe (2006). *Recommendation No. R (2006) 2 of the Committee of Ministers to Member States on the European Prison Rules (adopted 11 January 2006)*. Strasbourg, Council of Europe.
Council of Europe (1993). *3rd general report on the CPT's activities covering the period 1 January to 31 December 1992*. Strasbourg, Council of Europe, 1993 (CPT/Inf (93) 12).
Council of Europe (2001). *11th general report on the CPT's activities covering the period 1 January to 31 December 2000*. Strasbourg, Council of Europe, 2001 (CPT/Inf (2001) 16).

International Council of Nurses (1998). *Nurses' role in the care of detainees and prisoners*. Geneva, International Council of Nurses (http://www.icn.ch/psdetainees.htm, accessed 15 September 2006).

Norwegian Medical Association (2004). *Doctors working in prison: human rights and ethical dilemmas*. Oslo, Norwegian Medical Association (http://www.lupin-nma.net, accessed 15 September 2006).

Office of the United Nations High Commissioner for Human Rights (1957). *Standard Minimum Rules for the Treatment of Prisoners. Adopted by the First United Nations Congress on the Prevention of Crime and the Treatment of Offenders, held at Geneva in 1955, and approved by the Economic and Social Council by its resolution 663C (XXIV) of 31 July 1957 and 2076 (LXII) of 13 May 1977*. Geneva, Office of the United Nations High Commissioner for Human Rights (http://www.unhchr.ch/html/menu3/b/h_comp34.htm).

Prison Health Care Practitioners (1979). *Oath of Athens*. London, Prison Health Care Practitioners (http://www.prisonhealthcarepractitioners.com/Medical_ethics.shtml, accessed 15 September 2006).

United Nations (1966). *International Covenant on Economic, Social and Cultural Rights*. Geneva, Office of the United Nations High Commissioner for Human Rights (http://www.ohchr.org/english/law/cescr.htm, accessed 15 September 2006).

United Nations (1982). *Principles of Medical Ethics Relevant to the Role of Health Personnel, particularly Physicians, in the Protection of Prisoners and Detainees against Torture and Other Cruel, Inhuman or Degrading Treatment or Punishment. Adopted by General Assembly resolution 37/194 of 18 December 1982*. New York, United Nations.

United Nations (1990). *Basic Principles for the Treatment of Prisoners. Adopted and proclaimed by General Assembly resolution 45/111 of 14 December 1990*. New York, United Nations.

WHO Regional Office for Europe (1999). Mental health promotion in prisons: a consensus statement. In: *Mental health promotion in prisons: report on a WHO meeting, The Hague, the Netherlands, 18–21 November 1998*. Copenhagen, WHO Regional Office for Europe (http://www.euro.who.int/prisons/publications/20050610_1, accessed 15 September 2006).

WHO Regional Office for Europe (2003). *Declaration on Prison Health as a Part of Public Health*. Copenhagen, WHO Regional Office for Europe 2003 (http://www.euro.who.int/Document/HIPP/moscow_declaration_eng04.pdf, accessed 15 September 2006).

Further reading

Coyle A, Stern V (2004). Captive populations: prison health care. In: Healy J, McKee M, eds. *Accessing health care*. Oxford, Oxford University Press.

Tomascevski K (1992). *Prison health: international standards and national practices in Europe*. Helsinki, HEUNI.

3. Protecting and promoting health in prisons: a settings approach - *Paul Hayton*

Key points
- Prisoners tend to have poorer physical, mental and social health than the population at large.
- Prisons should regularly assess their population to ensure that health promotion and prevention programmes accurately address the needs of prisoners.
- Common problems such as bullying, mobbing and boredom make prison a difficult environment for promoting health but also a unique opportunity for reaching the hard to reach with important aspects of health promotion, health education and disease prevention. Prison can provide an important opportunity to reduce inequality in health.
- The needs of staff and prisoners must be considered together, especially in such areas as smoking cessation.
- A whole-prison or settings approach to promoting health draws on three key elements: 1) prison policies that promote health (such as a non-smoking policy); 2) an environment in a prison that is supportive of health; and 3) disease prevention, health education and other health promotion initiatives that address the health needs assessed within each prison.
- All staff members need to be made aware of their potential roles in promoting prisoners' health and trained and supported in these roles.
- A policy framework needs to be in place at the national level and the local level to support this type of work.

Introduction
In addition to providing health care, prisons should also provide health education, patient education, prevention and other health promotion interventions to meet the assessed needs of the prison population. Good health and well-being are key to successful rehabilitation and resettlement, and in turn this requires an environment in each prison that is supportive of health. This chapter offers guidance to help those working with prisoners:
- to build the physical, mental and social health of prisoners (and where appropriate staff) as part of a whole-prison approach;
- to help prevent the deterioration of prisoners' health during or because of custody; and
- to help prisoners adopt healthy behaviour that can be taken back into the community.

This chapter encourages the following as guiding principles:
- a whole-prison approach to health promotion in all prisons
- extended use of evidence-based health promotion in prisons
- disseminating information and good practice on health promotion and prevention.

Major problems that need to be addressed
In general, the prison populations in Europe come from the sections of society with

high levels of poor health and social exclusion. Prisoners tend to have poorer physical, mental and social health than the general population. Their lifestyles are more likely to put them at risk of ill health. Many prisoners have had little or no regular contact with health services before entering prison. Mental illness, drug dependence and communicable diseases are the dominant health problems among prisoners. Prisons should regularly assess the needs of their populations to ensure that health promotion and prevention programmes accurately address the needs of all prisoners.

A difficult challenge and a unique opportunity
Prison is an environment with special difficulty in the promotion of health. At the individual level, prison takes away autonomy and may inhibit or damage self-esteem. Common problems include bullying, mobbing and boredom, and social exclusion on discharge may be worsened as family ties are stressed by separation.

However, imprisonment is also a unique opportunity for all aspects of health promotion, health education and disease prevention.
- Prison offers access to disadvantaged groups who would normally be hard to reach. It is therefore a prime opportunity to address inequality in health by means of specific health interventions as well as measures that influence the wider determinants of health.
- Each prison has the potential to be a healthy setting: a single institution can address spiritual, physical, social and mental health and well-being.
- For the many prisoners who have led chaotic lifestyles prior to imprisonment, this is sometimes their only opportunity for an ordered approach to assessing and addressing health needs.

Prison is a home to one group of people and a workplace to another. Wherever possible, initiatives to promote the health of staff should be encouraged.

The health promotion needs of prisoners: examples of assessment
Assessment of health needs lies at the heart of successful interventions and useful outcomes. Health needs can be assessed by examining the epidemiological evidence and talking to stakeholders (including physicians and other health care staff but, importantly, all other staff who influence prisoners, such as education staff, and also prisoners themselves). The following section lists topics that are likely to be relevant in prisons across Europe, although it is far from exhaustive. Priorities must be created through a local process of assessing health needs.

All prisoners are likely to need:
- advice on preventing communicable diseases, including advice on avoiding sexually transmitted diseases, HIV infection and hepatitis, and advice on hepatitis B immunization;
- advice on high-risk lifestyles, including advice on avoiding drug overdose on leaving prison (needed by everyone because staff cannot identify everyone at risk); and protection against harm caused by smoking (including passive smoking);
- support in adopting healthy behaviour, including appropriate levels of physical activity and a balanced diet; and

- measures to promote mental health, including adequate time for association; a meaningful occupation (work, education, artistic activity and physical education); and contact with the outside world and help in maintaining family ties.

All prisoners should be considered to have these needs, although not all prisoners are necessarily at high risk. This is because staff has difficulty in identifying everyone at high risk and because all prisoners need information to reduce fear and stigma. These sorts of measures involve policy and practice not necessarily intended to affect health but with the potential to affect an individual's health and well-being.

Many prisoners are likely to need:
- training in psychological skills, including training in cognitive behavioural skills, activities to improve self-esteem, training for enhancing thinking skills and training in how to manage anger;
- health education and health-related education, including practical skills training, training in job search skills, parenting education, training in social and life skills, dietary advice and advice on physical activity and smoking; and
- specific health promotion interventions including access to a listener, buddy or the equivalent and support to give up drugs, alcohol or smoking.

Some prisoners are likely to need:
- patient education related to illnesses such as tuberculosis, including treatment options;
- immunization against tuberculosis, Pneumococcus infection or influenza;
- advice on specific conditions, such as minor illness, diabetes, epilepsy, asthma, menopause and sickle-cell disease; and
- access to cancer prevention and advice and services for early detection.

The whole-prison or settings approach and a vision for a health-promoting prison
Developing a whole-prison or settings approach to promoting health is important for improving the chances of intervention succeeding (Boxes 3.1 and 3.2).
The vision for a health-promoting prison is based on a balanced approach recognizing that prisons should be:
- safe
- secure
- reforming and health promoting
- grounded in the concept of decency and respect for human rights.

Human rights and decency are important foundations for promoting health because they underpin all aspects of prison life. Attaining the following measures creates a basis on which to promote health:
- treatment for prisoners that respects the law
- maintaining facilities that are clean and properly equipped
- providing prompt attention to prisoners' proper concerns
- protecting prisoners from harm
- providing prisoners with a regime that makes imprisonment bearable
- fair and consistent treatment by staff.

Box 3.1. Developing a whole-prison approach through a multidisciplinary team at a prison in England, United Kingdom

At HM Prison Risley (a medium security "training prison" for about 1000 men), a three-year health promotion strategy was developed, using a whole-systems approach to improving health and promoting health. A multidisciplinary team of committed staff and prisoners developed the healthy prisons project. The group also monitored the effectiveness of the projects.

Risley focused on the following areas:
- induction into the health care systems offered in the prison
- smoking cessation
- dads and families and high-quality family visits
- diet and nutrition
- hygiene
- mental health (with an emphasis towards offenders with mental disorders)
- sexual health and communicable diseases
- evening activities.

Box 3.2. A national approach: Prison Service Order 3200, a high-level policy instruction from HM Prison Service for England and Wales to encourage a whole-prison approach to creating a healthy prison

Prison service orders are mandatory for prison governors, who have to apply it in their own prison, and it states that (HM Prison Service for England and Wales, 2003):

Governors, working in partnership with the National Health Service, must ensure that ... they have included health promotion considerations adequately and explicitly within their local planning mechanisms .... The Health Promotion Section in the local plan must specifically address, as a minimum, needs in the five major areas:
1. *mental health promotion and well-being*
2. *smoking*
3. *healthy eating and nutrition*
4. *healthy lifestyles, including sex and relationships and active living*
5. *drugs and other substance misuse*

These areas of health and well-being should reflect a process of health needs assessment and not just healthcare needs assessment, and should involve a whole prison approach. Consultation should represent a wide variety of professional stakeholders, and prisoners must also be involved in this process. Prison Service Order 3200 has helped raise the profile of health promotion and the important contribution prisons can make to public health in England and Wales.

Fig. 3.1 A whole-prison approach to health promotion

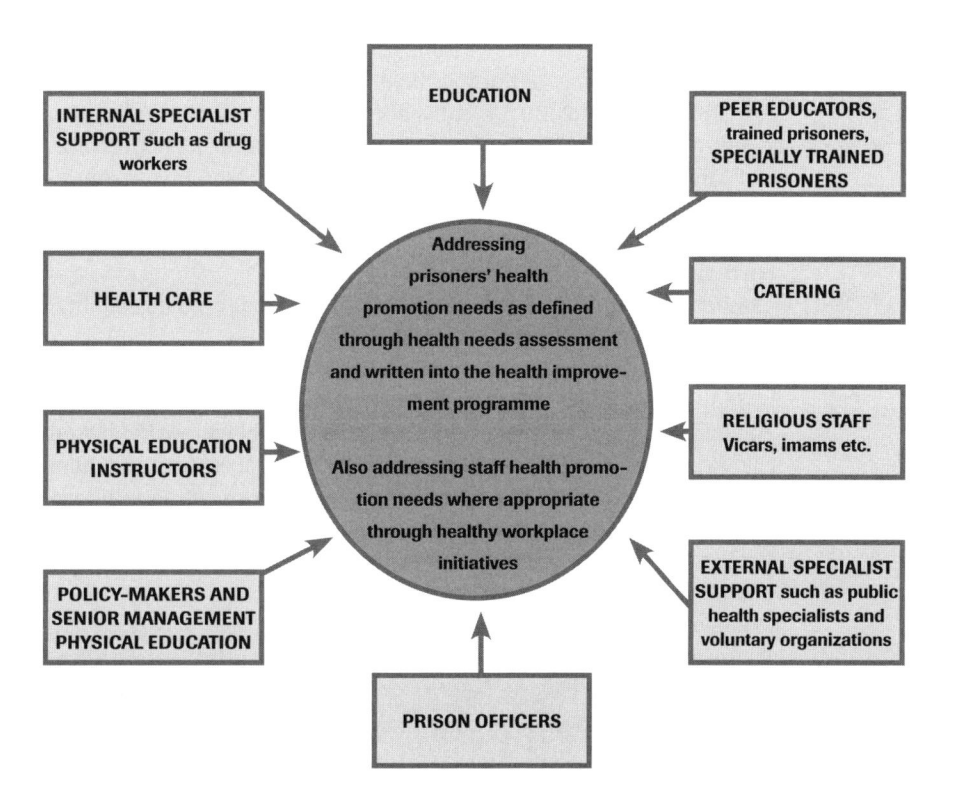

[Diagram: Central circle reads "Addressing prisoners' health promotion needs as defined through health needs assessment and written into the health improvement programme. Also addressing staff health promotion needs where appropriate through healthy workplace initiatives". Surrounding boxes: EDUCATION; PEER EDUCATORS, trained prisoners, SPECIALLY TRAINED PRISONERS; CATERING; RELIGIOUS STAFF Vicars, imams etc.; EXTERNAL SPECIALIST SUPPORT such as public health specialists and voluntary organizations; PRISON OFFICERS; POLICY-MAKERS AND SENIOR MANAGEMENT PHYSICAL EDUCATION; PHYSICAL EDUCATION INSTRUCTORS; HEALTH CARE; INTERNAL SPECIALIST SUPPORT such as drug workers.]

All managers, chief executives and governors in prisons across Europe and their staff can do the following.
- ensure that your prison promotes health and does not just provide health care;
- ensure that the responsibility of management for health promotion in your prison is clear, with clear line management responsibility, including teamwork implications;
- produce a prison policy statement on health promotion, and in your plans clarify any work commitments and resource implications and training required;
- adopt and implement the WHO Consensus Statement on Mental Health Promotion in Prisons (WHO Regional Office for Europe, 1999) – it is a good start for a whole-prison approach;
- adopt a whole-prison approach to health promotion as an integral part of prisons planning and practice – it should never be treated as solely a health care issue but should be recognized as part of the drive for decency and human rights in a prison;
- consider how you can monitor performance and evaluate progress; and
- consider as a priority the groups of prisoners and staff who may be most vulnerable to adverse health effects from prison and how to make these effects less harmful for them.

References
HM Prison Service for England and Wales (2003). *Prison Service Order 3200 – Health Promotion.* London, HM Prison Service for England and Wales (http://pso.hmprisonservice.gov.uk/PSO_3200_health_promotion.doc, accessed 15 September 2006).
WHO Regional Office for Europe (1999). Mental health promotion in prisons: a consensus statement. In: *Mental health promotion in prisons: report on a WHO meeting, The Hague, the Netherlands,* 18–21 November 1998. Copenhagen, WHO Regional Office for Europe (http://www.euro.who.int/prisons/publications/20050610_1, accessed 15 September 2006).

Further reading
Caraher M et al. (2002) Are health-promoting prisons an impossibility? Lessons from England and Wales. *Health Education,* 102:219–229.
Department of Health (2002). *Health promoting prisons: a shared approach.* London, Department of Health (http://www.dh.gov.uk/PublicationsAndStatistics/Publications/PublicationsPolicyAndGuidance/PublicationsPolicyAndGuidanceArticle/fs/en?CONTENT_ID=4006230&chk=AgAYAB, accessed 15 September 2006).
Ewles L, Simnet I (1999). *Health promotion: a practical guide.* London, Bailliere Tindall.
Hayton P, Boyington J (2006). Prisons and health reforms in England and Wales. *American Journal of Public Health,* 96:1730–1733.
Marshall T, Simpson S, Stevens A (2000). *Toolkit for health care needs assessment in prisons.* Birmingham, University of Birmingham (http://www.dh.gov.uk/assetRoot/04/03/43/55/04034355.pdf, accessed 15 September 2006).

4. Primary health care in prisons - *Andrew Fraser*

Key points
- Prison is a special setting for primary health care. All prison health services should strive to provide prisoners with health care equivalent to that provided in the community.
- The main purpose of health care is patient care, and prison health care is no different. Health professionals in prison also serve the courts and advise prison governors or directors. They should do so with the greatest possible involvement of their patients.
- Prisoners and health professionals each have rights and responsibilities. Professional groups should adhere to national standards of practice and to international rules and recommendations.
- Health professionals should understand and seek to minimize the negative effects of the experience of prison and use opportunities that prison can offer to benefit their patients.w
- Prison health services should understand the health needs of their patients and seek to meet their needs to the greatest extent possible within the available resources and norms for the country.
- Mental health, dependence problems and infections dominate most health needs of prisoners. Other types of chronic health conditions are also common and deserve attention.
- The primary care service should get to know their patients on admission, care for them during their stay and help to prepare them for release.
- Prison health services should understand the justice and health policy and the structures in which they work and seek to link with local services and resources, an especially important matter in managing people with severe mental illness.
- Every prison should have medical, nursing, dental, psychological and pharmacy services, with administrative support.
- Every prison should have access to health services at all hours.
- Every prison should maintain a system that accounts for its work, including its assets, resources, processes, key clinical challenges and outcomes, including critical incidents.
- Primary health care in prison is important for the well-being of the patients, all prisoners and the community, the effectiveness of prison services and the public health of the community.

Introduction
The health care of prisoners is an integral and essential part of every prison's work. Primary care is the foundation of prison health services.

Primary care is the most effective and efficient element of health care in any public health system (WHO, 1978) and as such, should be available to every prisoner. As described in more detail in chapter 2, prisoners have the same right to health care as everyone else in society.

The purpose of health care
In most respects, the purpose of health care in prison is the same as outside prison. The care of patients is its core function, and its main activities are clinical. A full primary care service, however, also includes elements of disease prevention and health promotion (Office of the United Nations High Commissioner for Human Rights, 1957).

As with primary care in the community, there are secondary duties. Prison health professionals may occasionally carry out other duties and services. They may provide reports to the court and for consideration of early release of prisoners, on general or specific health grounds. In most countries, these processes occur under the protection of laws and regulations. Unless there are exceptional circumstances, such as the potential for damage to a patient or to the interests of someone else mentioned in the report (a third-party interest), patients should be entitled to see and hold copies of reports and correspondence.

Despite the many similarities of health care between prison and the community, there are also differences. Prison brings loss of freedom, and this has many consequences for health care.

- The prisoners automatically lose the social component of health, including the loss of control of a patient's circumstances, the loss of family and familiar social support and a lack of information and familiarity with their surroundings.
- The environment of prison often poses a threat to mental well-being, especially a threat to a sense of personal security.
- In most circumstances, prisoners are unable to choose their professional health care team.
- Similarly, primary care teams in prison cannot select their patients.
- Neither the patient nor the health care team chooses the beginning and end of courses of treatment or of the clinician-patient relationship in general – this is largely decided by the courts.
- Generally, patients who are prisoners need a high level of health care.

Table 4.1 sets out the rights and responsibilities of patients and health care providers. The challenge for prisons is to minimize the negative effects of imprisonment on the health of prisoners and to work towards protecting health and enabling rehabilitation and care.

Table 4.1. Rights and responsibilities of patients and health care providers in prison

	Patients	**Primary care team**
Rights	Access to care	The means to practise health care to a standard equivalent to health care in the community
	Quality of care equivalent to that provided in public health services	Safety and security
	Confidential and private relationship	Freedom from threatening behaviour
	Humane treatment and respect	Mutual respect in relationship with patients
Responsibilities	Collaborate in treatment programmes	Act in interests of the patient above all
	Share personal health information with caregivers, to make well-informed decisions	Meet the requirements of the health professional and clinical team role
	Respect caregivers in a non-threatening and trusting relationship	Practise to the accepted general professional standards for the country
		Maintain confidentiality and privacy in the patient-clinician relationship
		Ensure professional competence
		Maintain good professional performance in areas of clinical practice required by patients
		Work well as a primary health care team in the interest of patients
		Work well with senior management and other staff in contributing to care programmes
		Work well with public health services in the community and hospitals

The experience of prison

All aspects of prisoners' life in prison affect their health and not simply the quality of health services provided.

In order to create the best conditions for good health and effective health care, prisons should adopt a whole-prison approach (for more detail, see chapter 3) and provide:
- a healthy environment and a culture of care and rehabilitation;
- an atmosphere in which prisoners feel safe in the company of other prisoners and staff;
- opportunities for prisoners to talk to other people in confidence;
- opportunities, through visits, to maintain family links;
- information about the prison routine;
- ways to keep loneliness and boredom to a minimum;
- adequate food, opportunities for exercise and access to fresh air; and
- sufficient privacy, adequate light, ventilation, heating (and sometimes cooling) and access to sanitation in the cell or barrack.

Prison staff and management should be aware of, and educated in basic health issues, particularly in what determines whether or not a prison environment promotes health. Staff should also be able to spot signs of serious illness, and experts in first aid and mental health should always be available to deal with crisis situations.

The components of primary care

The key components of a prison health service are contained in a section of the Standard Minimum Rules for the Treatment of Prisoners (Box 4.1), produced by WHO and the Office of the United Nations High Commissioner for Human Rights (1957). The remainder of this chapter is based on this authoritative source.

Box 4.1. Standard Minimum Rules for the Treatment of Prisoners
Medical services
22. (1) At every institution, there shall be available the services of at least one qualified medical officer who should have some knowledge of psychiatry. The medical services should be organized in close relationship to the general health administration of the community or nation. They shall include a psychiatric service for the diagnosis and, in proper cases, the treatment of states of mental abnormality.
    (2) Sick prisoners who require specialist treatment shall be transferred to specialized institutions or to civil hospitals. Where hospital facilities are provided in an institution, their equipment, furnishings and pharmaceutical supplies shall be proper for the medical care and treatment of sick prisoners, and there shall be a staff of suitable trained officers.
    (3) The services of a qualified dental officer shall be available to every prisoner.
23. (1) In women's institutions, there shall be special accommodation for all necessary prenatal and postnatal care and treatment. Arrangements shall be made wherever practicable for children to be born in a hospital outside the institution. If a child is born in prison, this fact shall not be mentioned in the birth certificate.
    (2) Where nursing infants are allowed to remain in the institution with their mothers, provision shall be made for a nursery staffed by qualified persons, where the infants shall be placed when they are not in the care of their mothers.
24. The medical officer shall see and examine every prisoner as soon as possible after his admission and thereafter as necessary, with a view particularly to the discovery of physical or mental illness and the taking of all necessary measures; the segregation of prisoners suspected of infectious or contagious conditions; the noting of physical or mental defects which might hamper rehabilitation, and the determination of the physical capacity of every prisoner for work.
25. (1) The medical officer shall have the care of the physical and mental health of the prisoners and should daily see all sick prisoners, all who complain of illness, and any prisoner to whom his attention is specially directed.
26. (2) The medical officer shall report to the director whenever he considers that a prisoner's physical or mental health has been or will be injuriously affected by continued imprisonment or by any condition of imprisonment.

The journey of primary care

At a minimum, primary care interventions are required at the times of highest risk to the health of prisoners, namely at the time of admission and before release, but are also needed to address health matters that arise during imprisonment.

- Every prisoner should be seen by a health professional at the time of reception and by a doctor soon after reception into prison (Box 4.2).
- Every prisoner should be assessed, or their health care reviewed, after a suitable period of settling into prison (Box 4.3).
- Primary health care in prison should be accessible to all prisoners when they request it, according to their needs. The needs of long-term prisoners should be

reviewed regularly and care and treatment goals agreed with the prisoner.
- Each patient should receive help in preparing them for release and should be put into contact with primary care services in the community.

Box 4.2. First assessment of each prisoner
On first assessment, the following questions should be examined:
1. Are the prisoners, as patients, a danger to themselves?
   (a) Do they have a serious illness, or are they withdrawing from an dependence or medication?
   (b) Are they at risk of self-harm or suicide?
2. Does the patient present a risk or a danger to others?
   (a) Do they have a disease that is easily transmitted that puts others at risk?
   (b) Is their mental state causing them to be a threat or are they likely to be violent?

Note: prison health professionals should assess the patient's risk to others on health grounds alone.

Box 4.3. Further assessment of each prisoner
Are immediate health problems (Questions 1 and 2 in Box 4.2) under control?
1. Do the problems require more detailed assessment and a treatment plan?
2. What is the past record and wider assessment of this person's health?
3. Does the person need specialist assessment, treatment plans or further reports?
4. Does the person need an integrated care plan for several problems – for instance, for mental health and dependence problems?
5. Who will take action on the care plans?
6. What can:
   (a) the patient do?
   (b) the health care team do?
   (c) secondary or specialist care contribute?
   (d) the rehabilitation team offer?
   (e) the prison generally do to support the patient's health?

Prison health care resources

Prisons should recognize that most prisoners need considerable health care. Adequate resources should be devoted to prison health care to provide prisoners with a standard of health care that is at least equivalent to that provided in the community outside. Further, taking advantage of the opportunity that imprisonment represents for the prisoners is important. Many come from marginalized and poor communities and are in poor health. Because prison health is public health, good health care in prison ultimately reduces the health risks to people in the community. All prison systems receive people who:

- are marginalized, poor, homeless or out of work, with mental health and dependence problems;
- have led a chaotic life, without access to proper and regular health care, and with several co-occurring health problems; and
- have health care needs requiring specialists from a number of disciplines, including dentistry, psychology, optometry and pharmacy.

Providing adequate primary care in prisons ideally leads to a narrowing of the health gap and to promoting equity in health by providing prisoners with access to care for known conditions that may not otherwise be available to them in the community (such as mental health care, dental care and management of long-term conditions); and by offering an opportunity to assess, detect and treat serious illnesses, especially mental health, infections and dependence problems.

Common problems encountered in primary care practice in prisons

Primary care in prisons has to deal with a very wide range of common problems (Box 4.4). Prisoners have a higher likelihood of almost any clinical problem compared with the general population. No conditions are unique to prison, but most conditions are more prevalent in prison. Some conditions can be influenced by prison conditions, often for the worse – such as air-borne infection, shared injecting equipment, anxiety, depression and other mental health problems.

Prison health care services must be able to deal with the following four priority areas:

- primary care
- mental health
- infections – especially tuberculosis, bloodborne viruses including HIV and skin conditions
- dependence, especially to drugs and alcohol.

Primary health care teams should be able to recognize and treat a range of chronic conditions. Common conditions among the prisoner population include epilepsy, lung and heart disorders and diseases and disorders of the reproductive system for women.

All health care services should be proficient in, or have ready access to, specialists in mental health care and drug dependence.

Box 4.4. Common problems in prison health care practice

Physical illness includes:
1. dependence (drugs, alcohol, tobacco);
2. infections;
3. dental disease; and
4. chronic disorders (lung disease, heart disease, diabetes, epilepsy, diseases of the reproductive system, cancer).

Mental health problems include:
1. low mood or self-confidence (self-esteem and dependence: drugs or alcohol)
2. anxiety
3. depression
4. severe mental disorders

Co-occurring problems include:
1. "vulnerable" people (learning disability, brain injury, learning difficulty, for instance resulting from autistic spectrum disorder or Asperger's syndrome or dyslexia; and
2. the nature of the sentence (harm against women, offences against children, bullying or recollection of being a victim of abuse).

Poor general condition includes:
1. hygiene
2. nutrition
3. mobility
4. personality disorder
5. physical and mental trauma and stress.

Building blocks for primary care in prison

The quality of primary health care in prison depends on many factors:
- the total resources available to the prison system;

- the state of development of primary health care in the community, including entitlement to dental, pharmacy and clinical investigation resources; and
- the development of mental health care in the community.

Within prison, factors that affect the quality of care include:
- the size of the prison population;
- the commitment of the governor or director to the health care of prisoners;
- whether the population is composed (primarily) of short- or long-stay prisoners;
- whether it is a prison for men or for women – women prisoners tend to have greater needs; and
- whether many of the prisoners come from vulnerable groups or are young adults or older people, who are likely to require more intervention.

Measuring performance in health care
The ability to measure performance depends on the resources allocated to prison health care and on the prison's capacity for recording information and for having achievable and recognized standards for good practice. It also reflects the state of the country's public health system.

Key areas for measuring performance are:
- facilities
- equivalent standards and arrangements with public health services
- knowing the needs of and capacity to meet the needs of prisoner-patients
- a supportive environment
- culture
- the time available for various tasks
- the quality of care
- focus on public health and health protection
- focus on health promotion
- health information systems
- links with public health services

Performance depends on adequate facilities and processes that allow prisoners easily to access health facilities. This is an important matter, dependent on security staff being able to escort prisoners and to provide safety and assurance for health care staff. In balance, facilities should allow for protection of confidentiality and privacy, with assessment and diagnostic facilities that match the skill and capacity of the public health service. More complex primary care services can include day care and inpatient accommodation. Facilities should be adequate to deliver care, including of sufficient size, clean, with natural light, good access for people with disabilities, and with meeting, reference and administrative facilities.

Equivalence to public health services – national prison health care should adhere to national codes of professional practice, standards of quality of care and regulatory matters. A positive aspect of demonstrating such equivalence is to use the same measures of quality assessment for prison services as:
- local public health services;
- national medical and professional institutions, colleges, academies and inde-

pendent prison inspection teams; and
- international organizations and comparable prison systems.

Prison health services require the capacity to record and understand the health needs of prisoners and to provide care with:
- resources that are sufficient to meet patient needs; and
- a prison culture that supports its health service and supports the access of prisoners to health care.

The prison director's leadership is vital in creating an environment in which prisoners and staff members value good health, feel safe and support each other. There should be a culture of respect and entitlement with:
- a humane health professional culture that respects patients' confidentiality and privacy and their right to health care equivalent to that sought after by the general public;
- an effective complaints system when things go wrong; and
- women must have an opportunity to see a woman physician or other health care attendant if they want to.

There must be sufficient time:
- to assess and treat patients;
- to meet as a health care team;
- to maintain professional development and networks of fellow professionals with common interests and to operate a method of appraisal that demonstrates staff learning in carrying out modern practice;
- to support active teaching and training programmes; and
- to have the capability to deliver good standards of care.

There must be quality of care.
- A medical practitioner working in prison should strive to have expertise, at least, in general medical practice, mental health, and dependence and infection control. These skills should be reflected in health care staff from other disciplines.
- Dental practitioners should be well trained in severe dental disease.
- Large establishments with specialist facilities – such as hospitals and day care – should have adequate staffing levels and skills to deal with seriously ill patients.
- Prisons that contain women or young people should employ practitioners with skills who are sensitive to particular conditions of these groups, including the care of young children.
- All health care professionals should be properly trained in the constraints of clinical practice in a prison, including the need for high standards of consistent practice, teamwork skills, good judgement in prescribing potentially addictive or mood-altering drugs and adherence to policy designed to uphold the confidence of vulnerable people who are patients in prisons.

The primary care service should have access or skills and capacity in public health and health protection matters. The Standard Minimum Rules for the Treatment of Prisoners also comment on the role of health care in this area (Box 4.5).

The Standard Minimum Rules for the Treatment of Prisoners also comment on the role of health care in this area (Box 4.5).
- Health care professionals should be educated, aware and demonstrate high standards of hygienic practice; capable of assessing cleanliness of patients and all prison facilities; and aware and capable of operating effective tuberculosis control, including auditing results.
- Effective control procedures are needed to limit the transmission of bloodborne viruses and sexually transmitted diseases.
- There should be a smoking control policy for health centres, prisoners and staff across the prison.
- Methods of reviewing critical incidents should be in place for key events such as deaths in custody, deaths following custody, suicide prevention programmes and people with serious mental illness.

Box 4.5. Excerpts from the Standard Minimum Rules for the Treatment of Prisoners
The medical officer shall regularly inspect and advise the director upon:
- the quantity, quality, preparation and service of food;
- the hygiene and cleanliness of the institution and the prisoners;
- the sanitation, heating, lighting and ventilation of the institution;
- the suitability and cleanliness of the prisoners' clothing and bedding; and
- the observance of the rules concerning physical education and sports, in cases where there is no technical personnel in charge of these activities.

The director shall take into consideration the reports and advice that the medical officer submits according to rules 25(2) and 26 (see Box 4.1) and, in case he concurs with the recommendations made, shall take immediate steps to give effect to those recommendations; if they are not within his competence or if he does not concur with them, he shall immediately submit his own report and the advice of the medical officer to higher authority.

A service should be developed that incorporates health promotion into the wider work of the prison, such as:
- encouraging people to acquire basic life skills;
- encouraging training towards employment and purposeful activity;
- locating suitable accommodation after release;
- encouraging participation in programmes to help people stop taking illegal and harmful drugs, smoking tobacco, and drinking excessive alcohol; and
- encouraging people to exercise regularly and to learn to prepare and enjoy foods that provide a balanced and nutritious diet.

Table 4.2. Key background factors important for health promotion for prisoners

Social, economic and life circumstances	Lifestyle	Health problems
Overcrowding	Smoking	Drugs and dependence
Ethnic diversity, language and religion	Drugs	Mental health
Disability, especially intellectual or developmental disability or brain disease	Alcohol	Dental health
Poverty	Diet	Infections
Poor hygiene or nutrition	Sexual health	Chronic conditions
Chaotic, unstructured lifestyle	Abusive relationships	
Poor educational attainment	Personality disorder	
Few assets or social capital		
History of past abuse		
Poor family capacity, parenting and supportive relationships		

Health services in prison should ensure high standards of maintenance of health records for patients, equivalent to best practice in the national public health service.
- There should be practical processes for recording, recalling and sharing clinical information to support the patient's care.
- There should be standard methods for reporting the work of health centres and accounting for the delivery of health care to the prison director, national prison services and outside organizations, using anonymous data extracted from health care records.
- There should be a complaints system for patients that is used both to correct apparent faults and to learn from patient experience.

Prison health care should have good links with public health services outside the prison, for many reasons:
- assuring the continuation of treatment for patients coming into prison;
- securing primary care services, mental health and dependence care and other continuing care following release from prison;
- ensuring access to specialist services;
- ensuring access to specialist public health help in the event of an incident or outbreak;
- ensuring that prison health care staff can access and benefit from education and training opportunities; and
- allowing for the sharing of clinical information between health professional staff for the purpose of direct patient care, in accordance with the patient's wishes and with good practice in ensuring confidentiality.

Conclusion
Health services in prison are primarily there for patients who are prisoners.

The senior clinician or manager is responsible for effective services on behalf of the prison director, often in partnership with the local public health service. Good services can profoundly affect the health of prisoners individually and collectively, the effective functioning of a prison system and the public health of the country. Routine systems of data collection and suitable clinical studies of challenges and problems should enable the primary care service in prison to describe, demonstrate and account for its service to patients who are in prison.

The setting of prison is special in many respects. It is an opportunity to deliver good primary care to a population whose health is often extremely poor and whose access to care is often hampered or denied.

References
Office of the United Nations High Commissioner for Human Rights (1957). *Standard Minimum Rules for the Treatment of Prisoners. Adopted by the First United Nations Congress on the Prevention of Crime and the Treatment of Offenders, held at Geneva in 1955, and approved by the Economic and Social Council by its resolution 663C (XXIV) of 31 July 1957 and 2076 (LXII) of 13 May 1977*. Geneva, Office of the United Nations High Commissioner for Human Rights (http://www.unhchr.ch/html/menu3/b/h_comp34.htm).
WHO (1978). *Primary health care. Report of the International Conference on Primary Health Care, Alma-Ata, USSR, 6–12 September 1978*. Geneva, World Health Organization (Health for All Series, No. 1; http://whqlibdoc.who.int/publications/9241800011.pdf, accessed 15 September 2006).

Further reading
Committee of Ministers of the Council of Europe (1998). *Recommendation No. R (98) 7 of the Committee of Ministers to Member States concerning the ethical and organisational aspects of health care in prison (adopted by the Committee of Ministers on 8 April 1998)*. Strasbourg, Council of Europe, 1998.
Committee of Ministers of the Council of Europe (2006). *Recommendation No. R (2006) 2 of the Committee of Ministers to Member States on the European Prison Rules (adopted 11 January 2006)*. Strasbourg, Council of Europe.
European Health Committee (1998). *The organisation of health care services in prisons in European Member States*. Strasbourg, Council of Europe.
Scottish Prison Service (2005). *Clinical governance audit framework*. Edinburgh, Scottish Prison Service.
Scottish Prison Service and NHS Education for Scotland (2005). *Competency framework for nursing staff working within the Scottish Prison Service*. Edinburgh, Scottish Prison Service and NHS Education for Scotland.
Scottish Prison Service/NHS Scotland (2006). *A guide to health needs assessment in Scottish prisons*. Edinburgh, Scottish Prison Service/NHS Scotland (http://www.sps.gov.uk/Default.asp?docid=1642, accessed 15 September 2006).

5. Prison-specific ethical and clinical problems -

Jean-Pierre Restellini

Key points
- Regardless of the circumstances, the ultimate goal of health care staff in prisons must remain the welfare and dignity of the patients.
- The results of medical examinations and tests undertaken in prison with consent as part of clinical care must be treated with the same respect for confidentiality as is normal under ethics in medical practice.
- In order to avoid as much as possible any confusion about the role of the doctor, between medical examinations and treatment in the care giving role, and other functions such as providing medical expertise (such as for forensic reports), the doctor should make it clear to the patient at the onset of the consultation that medical secrecy will not apply to the results of any medical examination and tests undertaken for the latter purposes.
- Regardless of security issues, the health care personnel should have unrestricted access at any time and any place to all detainees, including those under disciplinary measures.
- The health personnel should under no circumstances participate in enforcing any sanctions against prisoners or in the underlying decision-making process, as this will jeopardize any subsequent doctor-patient relationship.
- Medical personnel should not undertake any medical acts on restrained people (this includes handcuffs), except for people suffering from acute mental illness with potential for immediate serious risk for themselves or others.
- Doctors carrying out intimate body searches have to explain to the prisoners, before proceeding with the body search, that they are intervening purely as an expert and that their acts do not have a therapeutic or diagnostic purpose.
- During a hunger strike, doctors must avoid the risk that the detainees, the penitentiary or the judiciary authorities will instrumentalise their medical decisions.
- Doctors have a duty to document the physical signs and/or mental symptoms compatible with a detainee having been subjected to torture or cruel, inhuman and degrading treatment, and, taking into consideration the patients wishes, to report such acts through appropriate channels.
- The health service in a prison can potentially play a very important role in the fight against ill-treatment within the establishment and elsewhere. The physical and psychological examination performed on admission of a newcomer is particularly important in this respect.
- All health personnel working with detainees on an ongoing basis should have access to a specific training programme. It should address the issues of the specificities and inner workings of the different prisons, the handling of potentially dangerous or violent situations as well as the risks of ethical breaches specific to their activities as health care providers in prisons.

Introduction
Other chapters of this guide have already raised important issues relating to equivalence of care, confidentiality and informed consent of the patient detainee. This chapter will tackle other highly specific and sensitive health problems faced by the health personnel (as well as the penitentiary administration) in the practice of penitentiary medicine.

Health care staff in prison

Multiple loyalties

Doctors working in a prison are frequently torn between different loyalties. Their primary duty is to protect and promote the health of detainees and to ensure that the detainees receive the best possible care. This duty may, however, conflict with other priorities, notably those of the prison administration. In practice, the health care team is frequently obliged, despite its reticence, to take into account issues of order and security. Conversely, the security personnel may find it difficult to accept attitudes, beliefs and behaviour of health care staff that they perceive to conflict with prison rules and regulations.

Although it is not recommended, the prison doctor sometimes also officiates as a treating doctor for the security personnel (and sometimes even their families).[3] In such a context, the position of physicians is extremely complex since their duty is to take care simultaneously of people who are virtually in opposition if not in conflict.

This permanent state of tension can only be dealt with through regular meetings between the different professional bodies during which the necessary readjustments can be made. The exchanges during those encounters are even more essential as, in a large proportion of establishments, the acute lack of health personnel can force the penitentiary administrators to delegate certain health care-related tasks to security personnel.

Regardless of the circumstances, the ultimate goal to be followed by the health care staff must remain the welfare and dignity of the patients. It should be made plain to the patients, to the staff, and to the prison director that the prison health care staff's primary task is the health care of the inmates and that all work is carried out based on the strict medical and ethical principles of health care professionalism, independence and equivalence and confidentiality of care.

Parallel and conflicting activities

A doctor working in prisons may be called upon to perform two, somehow opposing roles. Firstly that of care giver to the detainee as patient, and secondly that of independent medical expert asked to provide medical evidence concerning the patient to a court or other judicial process. While the care-giver is concerned with the well-being of the individual patient, the doctor acting as a medical expert is asked to reveal medical information that would otherwise be confidential, in the interests of justice and in the service of the community. The common ethical rules establish that a doctor be one or the other. Only in case of crises or emergencies is it tolerated for the individual to combine these two functions.

However, in practice, penitentiary reality frequently obliges doctors to step out of their strict role as therapists. For instance, the judiciary or penitentiary authorities may ask physicians to vouch for a person's fitness to be detained or to prepare forensic reports in cases of allegations of ill treatment. Ideally such tasks should be

[3] The two types of activity of the doctor should preferably be clearly distinguished physically. It should be stipulated beforehand, for example, what percentage of the doctor's time is to be devoted to staff care and that two stocks of medication (detainees and staff) will be kept separately. Two separate consultation rooms would be best.

performed by an independent doctor from outside the prison system. If however the prison doctor has to perform such a task, the doctor charged with the task of examining a detainee as a medical expert should clearly inform the patient at the onset of the consultation that medical secrecy will not apply to the results of the medical examination and tests, in order to avoid confusing these two roles.

A penitentiary doctor may be asked to evaluate the threat to society a prisoner poses (with regard to a parole request or leave of absence). In such situations, the doctor must respond with extreme caution and clearly establish that his opinion can only be based on current assessment and must not be considered as definitive and predict future conduct. In such cases, since the prisoner may see the prison doctor as effectively playing a role in their release or continued detention, this has the potential to affect the doctor-patient relationship, and thus, again, it would be best if an independent medical opinion could be obtained.

Issues of conscience and serious ethical conflict
The multiple parameters affecting the work of prison doctors may run contrary to their personal convictions. It is therefore highly preferable to hire prison health care staff only on a voluntary basis and after preliminary specific training. In countries where the integration of prison health care services with the community health services has occurred, patients inside the prison are considered as simply another group within the wider community, and the health staff are thus expected to deliver services and care at the same level as that in the wider community.

In attempting to perform their duties according to the usual professional and ethical standards, doctors may face conflicts not only with decisions of the penitentiary administration, but also with local regulations and even national laws. In such cases, doctors should not remain in isolation but should ask their national professional organization (National Medical Association) for advice and, if needed, seek the opinion of colleagues working in other countries in the same field, including seeking the support of the World Medical Association[4].

Disciplinary measures
In any prisons, access to health care facilities may be arduous because of underlying security issues. This is particularly the case in disciplinary quarters and in maximum-security units. Penitentiary authorities often want to limit contact with certain detainees to a strict minimum.

However, regardless of the security issues, health care personnel should enjoy unrestricted access at any time and any place to all detainees, including those under disciplinary measures. The doctor in charge is responsible for ensuring that each detainee can, in practice, permanently exert his or her right of access to health care.

When penitentiary authorities decide to punish a detainee for breach of regulations, sanctions may take different forms. The health care personnel should never

---

[4] World Medical Association (WMA) was created to ensure the independence of physicians, and to work for the highest possible standards of ethical behaviour and care by physicians, at all times. For further information see www.mwa.net

participate in enforcing any sanctions or in the underlying decision-making process, as this is not a medical acts and thus to participate will jeopardize any subsequent doctor-patient relationship.

Doctors may often be approached when the sanction considered is disciplinary isolation (often termed solitary confinement). Disciplinary isolation has clearly been shown to be injurious to health, and moves to abolish the use of such practices have been promoted by the United Nations.[5] In cases where it is still enforced, its use should be limited to the shortest time possible. Thus, doctors should not collude in moves to segregate or restrict the movement of prisoners except on purely medical grounds, and they should not certify a prisoner as being fit for disciplinary isolation or any other form of punishment.

However, once a sanction is enforced, doctors must follow the punished detainee with extreme vigilance. It is well established that each disciplinary isolation event constitutes an important stress and risk (notably of suicide). Doctors must pay particular attention to this population of detainees and visit them regularly on their own initiative, as soon as possible after an isolation order has taken effect and thereafter daily, to assess their physical and mental state and determine any deterioration in their well-being. Doctors must immediately inform the penitentiary authorities each time a detainee presents a health problem.

Physical restraint
In prison, situations of extreme tension can erupt. In such cases, the penitentiary authorities can decide to use physical restraint against one or more detainees for the sole purpose of preventing harm to the prisoner themselves, or to other prisoners and staff. Again, the restraints must only be applied for the shortest time possible to achieve these purposes, and restraints can never be used as a form of punishment[6]. Since the decision to use restraints in situations of violence is not a medical act, the doctor must have no role in the process.

However, there may be instances where some form of restraint must be applied for medical reasons, such as acute mental disturbance in which the patient is at high risk of injuring themselves or others. The decision to use restraints for such purposes must be decided upon by the prison doctor and health staff alone, based purely upon clinical criteria, and without influence from the non-health prison staff.

Medical personnel should never proceed with medical acts on restrained people (this includes people in handcuffs), except for patients suffering from an acute mental illness with potential for immediate serious risk for themselves or others. Doctors should never agree to examine a blindfolded prisoner.

Intimate body searches
For security reasons, it may be necessary to search a detainee to ensure that he or she is not hiding anything in a natural body cavity. In many cases it may suffice to keep the prisoner under close surveillance and wait for the illicit object to be naturally expelled. Prison doctors and nurses should not carry out body searches, blood

---

[5] Basic Principles for the Treatment of Prisoners Adopted and proclaimed by General Assembly resolution 45/111 of 14 December 1990. Principle 7.
[6] Standard Minimum Rules. Rule 33.; and European Prison Rules (2006). Rule 68

or urine tests for drug metabolites or any other examinations except on medical grounds and with the consent of the patient. Vaginal, anal, and other intrusive bodily inspections are primarily a security, and not a medical, procedure, and thus should not form part of the duties of the healthcare providers of the prison. When, exceptionally, intimate body searches are deemed necessary external doctors should ideally be called in for such purposes. Otherwise, adequately trained security personnel of the same sex can undertake such examinations which must nevertheless be performed only according to established procedure which includes accountability, and in a manner compatible with the inherent dignity of the person.

Prisoners who stop eating or go on hunger strikes
Different reasons may motivate prisoners to stop eating.
- Religious issues: prisoners may stop eating as a part of specific religious festivals, or if food is served that is not prepared in accordance to religious precepts. The prison administration should deal with such issues and ensure that religious considerations are taken into account when preparing food for prisoners.
- Somatic problems: prisoners may stop eating because of somatic problems (such as dental problems, ulcers, obstructions of the digestive tract, very poor general health and fever). These should be resolved by putting into place the appropriate treatment.
- Mental disorders: prisoners may stop eating because of mental disorders, such as psychosis, poisoning delusion, major depressive disorders and anorexia nervosa. These prisoners should benefit from health care support of the kind they would receive in open society.
- Protest fasting: prisoners may stop eating with the intention of protesting to affect some change, either in regimens or privileges, or to obtain perceived or actual rights.

In the latter case, two sets of values clash:
- the duty of the state to preserve the physical integrity and life of those directly under its charge, notably people it has deprived of liberty; and
- the right of every individual to dispose freely of his own body.

Such situations are challenging for prison health care staff. Pressure is often brought to bear on the doctor, who should avoid the risk that the detainee, penitentiary or the judiciary authorities instrumentalise the medical decisions.

The most important guidance for prison doctors regarding hunger strikes is the Declaration on Hunger Strikes adopted by the 43rd World Medical Assembly in Malta in November 1991 (the Declaration of Malta[7]) and which was substantially revised in October 2006 (World Medical Association, 2006). To summarize the Declaration: doctors must obtain consent from the patients before applying any skills to assist them. Each person, including prisoners, has the right to refuse treatment as long as the following conditions are met.

The person is competent – in other words, does not suffer from mental disorders that alter their decision-making capacity. The doctor should interview every prison-

[7] World Medical Association Declaration on Hunger Strikers Adopted by the 43rd World Medical Assembly Malta, November 1991 and revised by the WMA General Assembly, Pilanesberg, South Africa, October 2006

er who is refusing food and ascertain the cause for refusal. Getting a second opinion from an independent psychiatrist as to soundness of mind is always wise in every case of food refusal.

The person is acting out of his or her own free will, meaning that he or she has not been subjected to external pressure (family, co-detainees or political group).

The refusal of treatment does not create a risk to others (this applies, for example, in the case of potentially contagious diseases such as tuberculosis).

When the fast appears to express a depressive state of mind in reaction to the judicial status of the detainee, with no obvious alteration of the decision-making capacity, doctors have to delicately choose a course of action. They have to keep in mind that the detainee does not wish to die in the vast majority of cases; quite to the contrary, the detainee wants to enjoy a better standard of living conditions. The patient frequently expects, without necessarily expressing it explicitly, that the doctor, who will invariably be called in if a hunger strike is maintained, will act as an intermediary and may act to protect him in this struggle.

In these situations, the medical approach should sometimes be frankly paternalistic. It should entail a persuasive discussion with the striking patients for them to accept at least a minimal caloric intake. Faced with a firm medical attitude, the depressed detainee may recover some hope and accept a normal healthy diet later.

Patients may ask for hospitalization to give their case more weight. In this situation, hospitalization unwarranted by clinical status should not appear as an indirect support to achieve aims. Nevertheless, early hospitalization may allow better follow-up of biological parameters. Further, a radical change of atmosphere could lead to a situation in which the detainee may choose to interrupt the hunger strike without losing face in front of comrades.

If the patient's position remains firm, based on "free will", to exert pressure through his body to modify a personal penal destiny or to conduct a political struggle, doctors should limit intervention to warning of the dangers to which strikers expose themselves by refusing to eat food.

The physician must visit patients regularly and, if the patient agrees, conduct regular follow-up examinations. These consultations should be held in a positive, personalized climate, and the physician should inform patients of the progressive decline of health. In this way, strikers can freely change their mind at any time and abandon the strike, having been duly informed of the worsening nature of the risks to which they are exposing themselves.

Occasionally strikers may ask to receive a certain type of diet, such as a hypercaloric concentrate in liquid form, rich in protein, vitamins and trace nutrients. It is usually best to grant the request. This prescription may protect the striker's health from irreversible damage. By lengthening the time of the fast, it can allow both the striking detainee and the authorities to propose a mutually acceptable solution for both parties in order to avoid lethal deadlock.

The doctor must keep the penitentiary and judicial authorities informed of the evolution of the health condition of the patient though regular and successive health reports. These carefully established and strictly objective health reports are part of the medical duty to a person in danger and allow the authorities to take more adequate decisions.

Clinical symptomatic aspects (in an initially healthy, young person)
In dry fasting, the individual refuses all solid or fluid intake. Death occurs in 4 to 10 days, depending on different factors such as:
- ambient temperature and humidity
- the striker's level of stress and physical activity

Alterations of the cardiac rhythm usually cause death.

In total fasting, the individual only consumes clear water, with no other intake of nutrients.

In theory, the reserves of the human body should allow a person to survive between 75 to 80 days without absorbing a single calorie. Nevertheless, serious, sometimes deadly, clinical disorders may appear after only 40 days of complete fasting due to problems in the nervous system or cardiovascular system caused by vitamin depletion or major electrolyte imbalances.

The usual clinical evolution of a hunger strike in a healthy, young patient who continues to drink water proceeds as follows.

First week
Sensation of hunger and fatigue. Occasional, possible abdominal cramping.

Second and third week
Increasing weakness, accompanied by dizziness, making the upright position difficult to maintain. Progressive disappearance of the feelings of hunger and thirst. Permanent sensation of chilliness.

Third and fourth week
Progressive worsening of the symptoms mentioned above. Slowing down of intellectual faculties.

Fifth week
Alteration of consciousness (from mild confusion to stupor and sleepiness, apathy and anosognosia, followed by anomalies of ocular movements (initially uncontrollable movements followed by paralysis). Generalized lack of motor coordination with a notable difficulty in swallowing. Diminishing vision and hearing, leading to loss of vision and hearing. Sometimes diffuse haemorrhaging.

Death can occur abruptly either due to cardiac rhythm alterations or several hours after the induction of a comatose state due to hypoglycaemia.

Today most strikers follow dietary fasts with absorption of certain vitamins, trace minerals and some food (sweet drinks, candy or small amounts of various foods). This type of hunger strike allows one to "hold on" for several months, even if a prolonged hunger strike poses a substantial risk of permanent nervous system damage: specifically Wernicke syndrome, a collection of nervous system symptoms characterized by a state of mental confusion and marked problems of equilibrium.

In practice, because many different factors affect a fast (such as the type of fasting, detention conditions (temperature, humidity) and mental stressors), determining medically the risk and timing of death is practically impossible.

However, certain medical factors can predispose to the rapidly fatal evolution of a fast. Major ones include heart disease (especially coronary heart disease) and renal insufficiency. Relative ones include diabetes, especially if type 1, gastritis, gastric or duodenal ulcers can manifest as problems during the first 10 days of the fast.

Feeding should never be forced in prison. Such a procedure can only be justified if a serious mental disorder affects the decision-making capacity of the patient. Generally, however, when a hunger strike is the logical expression of a lucidly thought out struggle and not a pathological response by a severely depressed patient considering suicide, prison doctors have to respect the expressed will of the patient and limit themselves to the position of medical counsellor. The revised Declaration of Malta specifically states that forcible feeding is never ethically acceptable, and goes further in stating that feeding accompanied by threats, coercion, force or use of physical restraints is in the huge majority of cases a form of inhuman and degrading treatment. It is clear from this statement that medical personnel cannot ethically participate in a procedure that is in itself a form of ill-treatment.

Torture and inhumane or degrading treatment
Medical personnel seriously violate the rules of medical ethics if they:
- in any way assist in (even by merely being present) sessions of torture or advise the torturers;
- provide facilities, instruments or substances to that effect;
- certify that a prisoner is able to withstand a torture session; or
- weaken the resistance of the victim to torture.

However, the health service in a prison can potentially play a very important role in the fight against ill treatment within the establishment and elsewhere (specifically police stations). In the context of medical consultations, people sometimes show physical signs or even mental symptoms compatible with having been subjected to torture or other forms of cruel, inhuman or degrading treatment.

In light of these facts, the physical and mental examination performed on admission of a newcomer is particularly important.

During a physical examination (and most specifically the one performed upon arrival), any trace of violence compatible with torture must be duly noted and registered, both in the personal file of the detainee as well as any general register listing traumatic lesions. Equally, any psychological or psychiatric disturbances that may also indicate that the person has been subjected to any form of ill-treatment must be recorded. Such information must be automatically transmitted with no delay to the prison or judiciary surveillance authorities. Detainees can obtain a copy of their medical report at any time.

However, the simple fact of being identified by the health care services as bearing traces of traumatic lesions or mental symptoms compatible with torture can trigger measures of reprisal against the victim. In order to best protect patients from this risk of retaliation, doctors must formally inform patients that they are going to report to the competent authority the evidence they have gathered during the consultation. If the patients fear that they will be subjected to reprisal, they may decide not to divulge how the lesions were inflicted and even lie about them.

In their report, doctors must clearly distinguish between the allegations (circumstances of the physical or mental trauma as described by the patient) and the complaints (subjective sensations experienced by the patient) from the clinical and para-clinical objective findings (mental state; size, location, aspect of the lesions, X-rays, laboratory results, etc.). If the doctors' training and/or experience allow it, they must indicate whether the patients' allegations are compatible with their own clinical findings.

Capital punishment
Health professionals should never be complicit in any way (even by their presence) to capital punishment, should not be involved in examining the detainee immediately before the execution, nor in confirming death and should not issue the death certificate.

Conclusions
This chapter indicates the indispensable qualities, both human and professional, that are required to work correctly and ethically as a member of the health services in such a complex environment.

All health personnel providing care to detainees on an ongoing basis should have access to a specific training programme. It should address all the issues addressed in this chapter, including the particularities of working in different prisons, the handling of potentially dangerous or violent situations and the risks of ethical breaches specific to their activity as a health care provider in prison.

Reference
World Medical Association (2006). *Declaration of Malta on Hunger Strikers*. Adopted by the 43rd World Medical Assembly Malta, November 1991 and editorially revised at the 44th World Medical Assembly Marbella, Spain, September 1992, and revised by the WMA General Assembly, Pilanesberg, South Africa, October 2006

Further reading
Antonovsky A (1979). *Health, stress and coping: new perspectives on mental and physical well-being*. San Francisco, Jossey-Bass.
Augestad LB, Levander S (1992). Personality, health and job stress among employees in a Norwegian penitentiary and in a maximum-security hospital. *Work & Stress*, 6:65–79.

Bögemann H (2004). *Gesundheitsförderung in totalen Institutionen.* Oldenburg, BIS-Verlag (Schriftenreihe "Gesundheitsförderung im Justizvollzug", Band 10).

Committee of Ministers of the Council of Europe (2006). *Recommendation No. R (2006) 2 of the Committee of Ministers to Member States on the European Prison Rules (adopted 11 January 2006).* Strasbourg, Council of Europe.

Council of Europe (1993). *3rd general report on the CPT's activities covering the period 1 January to 31 December 1992.* Strasbourg, Council of Europe, 1993 (CPT/Inf (93) 12).

Council of Europe (2001). *11th general report on the CPT's activities covering the period 1 January to 31 December 2000.* Strasbourg, Council of Europe, 2001 (CPT/Inf (2001) 16).

Coyle A (2002). *A human rights approach to prison management: handbook for prison staff.* London, International Centre for Prison Studies.

European Health Committee (1998). *The organisation of health care services in prisons in European Member States.* Strasbourg, Council of Europe.

Gerstein L, Topp H, Correl G (1987). The role of the environment and person when predicting burnout among correctional personnel. *Criminal Justice and Behavior*, 14:352–369.

Goffman E (1961). *Asylums. Essays on the social situation of mental patients and other inmates.* Harmondsworth, Penguin.

Office of the United Nations High Commissioner for Human Rights (1999). Health professionals with dual obligations. In: *Manual on the Effective Investigation and Documentation of Torture and Other Cruel, Inhuman or Degrading Treatment or Punishment (Istanbul Protocol).* Geneva, Office of the United Nations High Commissioner for Human Rights.

Penal Reform International (1995). *Making standards work: an international handbook on good prison practice.* The Hague, Penal Reform International.

United Nations (1982). *Principles of Medical Ethics Relevant to the Role of Health Personnel, particularly Physicians, in the Protection of Prisoners and Detainees against Torture and Other Cruel, Inhuman or Degrading Treatment or Punishment. Adopted by General Assembly resolution 37/194 of 18 December 1982.* New York, United Nations.

Whitehead J, Lindquist C (1986). Correctional officer job burnout. A path model. *Journal of Research in Crime and Delinquency*, 23:23–42.

WHO Regional Office for Europe (1999). Mental health promotion in prisons: a consensus statement. In: *Mental health promotion in prisons: report on a WHO meeting, The Hague, the Netherlands, 18–21 November 1998.* Copenhagen, WHO Regional Office for Europe (http://www.euro.who.int/prisons/publications/20050610_1, accessed 15 September 2006).

Wool R, Pont J (2006). Prison health. *A guide for health care practitioners in prisons.* London, Quay Books.

World Medical Association (1975). *Declaration of Tokyo: Guidelines for Medical Doctors Concerning Torture and Other Cruel, Inhuman or Degrading Treatment or Punishment in Relation to Detention and Imprisonment.* Helsinki, World Medical Association.

World Psychiatric Association (1996). *Declaration on Ethical Standards for Psychiatric Practice.* Chêne-Bourg, World Psychiatric Association.

6. Communicable diseases - *Dumitru Laticevschi*

Key points
- Prisoners are at great risk of contracting communicable diseases: they have no control over their environment, and the combination of factors of transmission – agents, hosts and routes of transmission – is much less favourable in prisons than it is outside.
- Communicable diseases result from interactions between agents and hosts but are influenced by factors such as financing of health care services and prison management practices.
- Communicable diseases in prisons cannot be successfully controlled through isolated clinical interventions. For the benefit of prisoners, prison staff and society in general, concern for health must be integrated into broader public policies that affect prisons.
- Cost-effective public health interventions with a solid evidence base exist for controlling communicable diseases.

Introduction

As far back as in the antiquity, people understood that public sanitation can decrease the spread of diseases. The Roman state supported the provision of food, supplies of clean water and bathing facilities. When increasing trade and mobility of populations led to the growth, overcrowding and unhealthiness of the medieval cities, isolation of the sick and quarantines for those coming from outside the city who had suffered potential exposure offered an efficient instrument for controlling disease to the cities that were able to consistently enforce such measures. In more recent times, the discovery of vaccines and antibiotics has brought about spectacular changes, leading, among other things, to the eradication of smallpox and a drastic reduction of infant mortality. Yet despite the long history of collecting evidence and the recent advances in the health sciences, worldwide, in the 21st century infectious diseases remain the leading cause of death. The main reason why individuals are vulnerable is that the source of infection usually lies outside the individual. Exposure to the environment or to other infected individuals is the key factor in transmission.

Prisoners are at particular risk, as they have virtually no control over their environment and usually have no choice over the density and composition of their surroundings. The combination of factors of transmission – agents, hosts and routes of transmission – is much less favourable in prisons than it is usually outside (Fig. 6.1).

Fig. 6.1. Interaction of factors causing communicable diseases in prisons

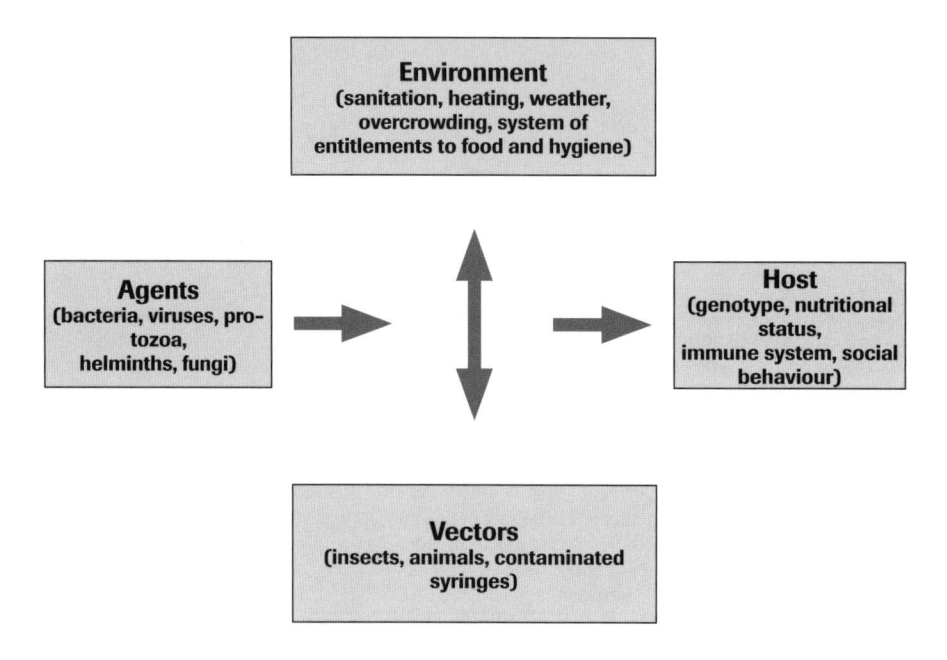

```
                    ┌─────────────────────────┐
                    │      Environment        │
                    │ (sanitation, heating,   │
                    │  weather, overcrowding, │
                    │  system of entitlements │
                    │  to food and hygiene)   │
                    └───────────┬─────────────┘
                                ↕
┌──────────────────┐            │           ┌──────────────────┐
│     Agents       │            │           │       Host       │
│ (bacteria,       │ ──→        │     ──→   │ (genotype,       │
│  viruses, pro-   │            │           │  nutritional     │
│  tozoa,          │            │           │  status, immune  │
│  helminths,      │            │           │  system, social  │
│  fungi)          │            │           │  behaviour)      │
└──────────────────┘            │           └──────────────────┘
                                │
                    ┌───────────┴─────────────┐
                    │        Vectors          │
                    │ (insects, animals,      │
                    │  contaminated syringes) │
                    └─────────────────────────┘
```

Agents (bacteria, viruses, protozoa, helminths and fungi) are a necessary link in the chain of infection. The vast majority of the prison population consists of people from poor and marginalized communities with little access to health services. Because of behaviour, life circumstances and material conditions, infectious agents are more prevalent among these people.

A typical prisoner is more likely to be a disempowered individual with a history of disease exposure, drug use and alcohol consumption. He or she is more likely to experience overcrowded premises both before and after imprisonment and can be exposed to diseases through food and water.

Neglected chronic diseases, anatomical defects, coexisting infectious and non-infectious diseases, a history of inconsistent antibiotic use, high dosage and prolonged duration of exposure and poor nutritional status negatively influence the frequency of occurrence and severity of disease in prisons.

In the crowded and often insalubrious prison environment, infectious agents can spread in a variety of different ways: directly – through touching, sexual intercourse, direct droplet projection from a coughing individual or contact with soil – or through several indirect transmission mechanisms: carrier-borne transmission can occur through food, water, clothing, tattooing equipment or contaminated syringes; airborne transmission can occur through the aerosols created in the large, poorly ventilated and scarcely heated rooms; and vectors can be transmitted through flies, mosquitoes and ticks.

Disease prevention in prisons can be organized at three levels.
- At the individual level, the health staff members usually provide clinical interventions – such as administering antibiotics to prevent infection of wounds or treating scabies to prevent bacterial complications. However, substantial health services in prisons are delivered in lay settings as self-care or as care for the peers. Care should be taken to avoid blaming individuals for their behaviour leading to disease, since individuals often do not fully control the circumstances.
- At the institutional level, safe methods of searching and screening can prevent exposure to bloodborne diseases, or administrative arrangements for ventilating the indoor spaces can decrease the transmission of tuberculosis.
- At the population level, health-promoting interventions are organized from a public health perspective and can include regulating the quantity and quality of food, adopting standards for quality of water or indoor air and implementing policies for exchange of syringes.

To prevent the spread of communicable diseases, the weakest links of the chain agent–transmission–host have to be targeted (Fig. 6.1). For example, chlorinating water destroys some agents; promoting the use of condoms removes the contact needed for transmission; using repellents, disinfectants and protective clothing targets the vectors; and vaccination immunizes the host.

In choosing the most appropriate strategy, policy-makers need to consider the risks associated with the disease, the feasibility of interventions, the costs and benefits of the interventions and equity considerations. Because of the particular circumstances of prisons, some approaches may be more difficult to apply.

Prisons in general and prison health in particular are not always high on the agenda of politicians, but the threat of transmission of infectious diseases in prisons and ultimately from prisons to general society demonstrates the importance of ensuring better access to health care and health promotion in prisons. Prisons represent both a challenge and an opportunity in controlling the spread of infectious diseases: a challenge because the conditions in prison often increase the risk of transmission, but also an opportunity, because many individuals have much better access to health services in prison than they normally do outside the prison. In addition, the prison population is compact and not excessively mobile, which makes efforts to screen for infectious diseases relatively easier. Finally, achieving adherence to treatment can be easier in prison than outside.

Bloodborne diseases

Bloodborne agents are those that are present in human blood and that can cause disease in other humans who are exposed to blood or blood products. The most relevant (but not the only) bloodborne agents include hepatitis B virus, hepatitis C virus and human immunodeficiency virus (HIV). In prisons, both health care workers and the security staff can be exposed to blood and other body fluids through sharps injuries (needle sticks and other), mucous membrane exposure and skin exposure. The general precaution measures for preventing bloodborne viruses in prisons include the following.

Health care and security staff need:
- to treat every subject as a potential host of bloodborne agents
- to avoid directly handling contaminated materials
- to wear gloves for all procedures in which exposure to blood or other body fluids is likely.

Health care staff need:
- to cover all cuts with waterproof dressings;
- to use improvised absorbent barriers (such as towels and handkerchiefs) when handling actively bleeding wounds;
- to thoroughly clean and sterilize instruments contaminated with blood; and
- to use effective disinfectants (such as bleach).

The administration must ensure that adequate equipment is available to protect security staff; that health care staff have the equipment needed to make health care procedures safe for them and for the prisoners; and that prisoners have access to the tools that will protect them from contracting infections (and ultimately, make prisons a safer place for prison staff), such as bleach to allow for disinfection of sharp objects and needle and syringe programmes.

The following section explains in more detail how the risk of intravenous transmission of bloodborne viruses and transmission through tattooing and piercing can be reduced.

Tattooing and piercing
Although tattooing is prohibited in prisons in many countries, it is a very common activity. Tattoos are often applied in unclean conditions using pencils, pens, straight pins or needles. The pigments injected can include carbon, soot, mascara, charcoal and dirt. Dirty tattooing equipment can act as an efficient vehicle for transmitting bloodborne infections. Tattooing is associated with the risk of acquiring HIV, hepatitis B virus, hepatitis C virus and tetanus. The tattoo dyes can cause allergic reactions. Rarely, when hygiene is very poor, and the diseases are widespread, tuberculosis and syphilis can be transmitted if urine and saliva are used in the tattooing process.

Piercing is also prevalent in many prisons. The body parts that are most commonly pierced are the earlobe and ear cartilage, eyebrow, lip, nose, tongue, nipple, navel and genitals. The body jewels are inserted in the holes left by needles in the body parts. In some prison cultures, metal balls are frequently inserted into the foreskin or it is impregnated with ointments to increase the diameter. Biologically inert metals such as surgical steel or gold are rarely available to prisoners, which increases the risk of infections and allergic reactions.

Preventing the transmission of bloodborne diseases through tattooing requires efforts at three levels.
- At the individual level, tattooists should wash their hands and use gloves. They should have the means to sterilize the equipment between uses on different prisoners – ideally, sterile tattoo needles should be used only once and then disposed of in safe containers. The remaining tattoo ink must always be thrown

away after procedures. The site of a tattoo needs to be cared for similarly to a superficial burn: the area must be kept clean and moisturized until the tattoo is completely healed.
- At the level of the institution, safe tattoo rooms can be set up, and conditions for sterilizing equipment can be offered to reduce the transmission of bloodborne diseases. However, facilities for safe tattooing are rarely available in prisons. In the absence of such facilities, inmates should reserve clean areas with good illumination for tattooing (or piercing).
- At the population level, clean tattooing equipment should be available to prisoners, and they should be able to set up safe tattoo rooms, but the degree to which this is possible depends on how receptive prison administrations and ministries responsible for prisons are to public health arguments.

Intravenous transmission
Blood transfusions are associated with the highest risks of transmission of bloodborne infections. However, blood safety measures – selecting donors and screening donated blood – have drastically reduced the probability of acquiring bloodborne infections through transfusions.

Sharing syringes for injecting drug use is also a very efficient way of transmitting bloodborne diseases. Despite efforts to keep drugs from entering prisons, injecting drug use is common in many prisons and creates a great risk factor for transmission of bloodborne infections. Because smuggling injecting equipment into prisons is much more difficult than smuggling drugs, often only a few syringes circulate in prison, which increases the likelihood that many people will inject using the same syringe. When a syringe enters the vein, the plunger is pulled back to ensure that the needle is in the vein. Some of the blood that enters into the syringe may remain in it and be injected by the next user. Transmission is caused by the exchange of blood. The injecting drug user who never shares syringes will not get HIV or other bloodborne infections from syringes.

Prevention is based on blocking transmission caused by using contaminated syringes. At the population level, adopting pragmatic policies to reduce risk creates the most favourable conditions for preventing transmission. If such policies are in place, the institutions can promote safe injecting practices by interventions ranging from health education to needle and syringe programmes. The individual drug user should avoid sharing injecting equipment and, when needle and syringe programmes are available, take part. If clean needles and syringes are not available, bleach should be used to reduce the risk of transmission, but this will not eliminate the risk. The high concentration of hepatitis B virus and hepatitis C virus in the bloodstream and their ability to survive outside the body make them much easier to contract than HIV. To prevent infection with hepatitis B virus and hepatitis C virus, injecting drug users should avoid sharing any part of their injecting materials, including syringe, cotton, water and cooker.

Tuberculosis
Tuberculosis is caused by Mycobacterium tuberculosis. These bacteria are spread through the air and attack primarily the lungs. The source is the person with active pulmonary tuberculosis who spreads the Mycobacterium tuberculosis by airborne

particles, when coughing, sneezing, speaking or singing. Prisons are often overcrowded and poorly heated. To prevent the loss of heat, inmates often seal the windows, which creates the perfect environment for Mycobacterium tuberculosis to persist in the air. Persons who share the room with people with active tuberculosis are at the greatest risk of infection.

Most individuals who inhale tuberculosis bacteria and become infected have no symptoms and do not feel sick. Mycobacterium tuberculosis stays alive in their bodies but stops growing. This situation is called latent infection. Most people who have latent tuberculosis infection never develop active tuberculosis. But when the immune system cannot stop the bacteria from growing, the Mycobacterium tuberculosis starts multiplying, causing active tuberculosis. People infected with HIV have very weak immune systems, which increases their vulnerability. The prevalence of HIV in prisons is higher than in the general population, which creates an additional burden for tuberculosis control programmes. Substance abuse and low body weight, both prevalent in prison, can also weaken a person's immune system.

The individual behaviour of people with tuberculosis can significantly reduce the spread of tuberculosis:
- most importantly, tuberculosis drugs must be taken regularly;
- covering the mouth with a tissue when coughing, sneezing or laughing is also important;
- people with active tuberculosis should not go to places where contact with healthy people is possible; and
- windows should be opened frequently so that rooms can be ventilated adequately.

Remember that tuberculosis is spread through the air. Despite widespread misconceptions, people cannot get infected through handshakes, sitting on toilet seats or sharing dishes and utensils with someone who has tuberculosis.

Pulmonary tuberculosis can cause such symptoms as:
- coughing for more than two weeks
- coughing up sputum or blood
- chest pain
- weakness and fatigue
- weight loss
- fever
- night sweating.

Institutional measures to prevent the spread of tuberculosis include schedules for ventilating living areas, measures to ensure good heating (while avoiding sealing windows) and allowing prisoners to spend enough time outside. Support for case finding – such as by referring prisoners with symptoms to health care workers – can lead to earlier treatment, reducing the amount of time people who are infectious spend with other prisoners, and can therefore be an efficient measure for controlling tuberculosis.

The fact that tuberculosis can be cured with correct treatment led to the most potent interventions – the ones that take into account the population perspective. Mathematical modelling has shown that identifying at least 75% of the infectious cases and curing at least 85% of them will sharply reduce the rate of transmission in the population – to the extent that this effectively controls disease. These are the classical objectives of tuberculosis control under the strategy recommended by WHO (for further information, see chapter 8).

Ideally, tuberculosis control in prisons should be integrated into a country's national tuberculosis control programme, but where this is not possible, the prison tuberculosis services can be strengthened alone. High-quality treatment with a full spectrum of tuberculosis drugs will positively affect both individuals and the prison population as a whole without significant risk of resistance, even in the extreme case when some people cannot complete their course because they are released before treatment ends.

The diagnosis is based on staining and direct microscopy of sputum. Mass X-ray screening is justified in the prison population, but it needs to be complemented with screening for symptoms and with passive case-finding.

WHO case definitions
To avoid improper treatment in people who have previously been treated (and hence, to reduce the possibility of selecting resistance), to ensure efficient use of resources and to reduce the number of side effects by avoiding excessive doses, WHO recommends that the standard treatment regimens be matched to the diagnostic category of each case of tuberculosis. The case definitions are determined by the site of tuberculosis, the result of sputum smear microscopy, the severity of tuberculosis and the history of previous treatment for tuberculosis.

Usually, after taking drugs for a few weeks, people with tuberculosis feel good and may stop being infectious. This has important consequences – when people with tuberculosis are not infectious and do not feel sick, they can function the same way as before they had active tuberculosis. Unfortunately, the diagnosis of tuberculosis often sticks to individuals long after they stop being infectious, causing unjustified stigma, distracting the attention from the unknown active cases of tuberculosis or from the people with tuberculosis being treated who are still infectious.

The tuberculosis drugs can occasionally cause side effects. Some of the more serious are: loss of appetite, nausea and vomiting; yellowish skin or eyes; fever for three or more days; abdominal pain; skin rash; bleeding easily; changed vision; ringing in the ears; and hearing loss.

Although the clinical situation improves rapidly, tuberculosis bacteria die slowly in the body of the person with tuberculosis. At least six months is required to complete the treatment.

Treatment outcomes
Incomplete treatment may lead to relapses and to the development of resistance to tuberculosis drugs. This means that the medicine can no longer kill the bacteria. Sometimes the bacteria become resistant to the two most potent tuberculosis

drugs: isoniazid and rifampicin. This situation is called multidrug-resistant tuberculosis and represents a very serious problem. Multidrug-resistant tuberculosis is treated with second-line tuberculosis drugs that are less effective than the usual tuberculosis drugs and may cause more side effects.

To ensure that the treatment takes place without interruption, most tuberculosis control programmes have introduced directly observed therapy (DOT). The drugs are thus taken while the health care worker watches the intake. The progress of treatment is measured after the initial phase at the end of the second month by microscopy of sputum and then again in the continuation phase and at the end of treatment.

An important managerial feature of the WHO strategy for controlling tuberculosis is that treatment outcomes (Table 6.1) are registered in a way that enables cohort analysis.

Table 6.1. WHO definitions of the outcome of tuberculosis treatment

Cure	Patient who is sputum smear-negative in the last month of treatment and on at least one previous occasion
Treatment completed	Patient who has completed treatment but who does not meet the criteria to be classified as a cure or failure
Treatment failure	Patient who is sputum smear-positive at five months or later during treatment
Death	Patient who dies for any reason during the course of treatment
Default	Patient whose treatment was interrupted for two consecutive months or more
Transfer out	Patient who has been transferred to another recording and reporting unit and for whom the treatment outcome is not known

Sexually transmitted infections

A prison population affected by sexually transmitted infections may expect an increase in the number of cases of HIV infection: the sexually transmitted infections that disrupt the integrity of the skin or mucous membranes can bleed easily, thereby increasing a person's infectiousness and susceptibility to HIV. Further, sexually transmitted infections are an important predictor of HIV infection because they indicate the presence of behaviour associated with the transmission of HIV. The best way to prevent sexually transmitted infections is to avoid sexual contact altogether, but this is not realistic for many prisoners, most of whom are in their sexually active years and some of whom may be subjected to various forms of sexual abuse. However, prisoners can be encouraged to learn how to prevent sexually transmitted infections and the common symptoms of sexually transmitted infections and seek health care as soon as they notice any symptoms.

HIV

HIV is found in blood but also in semen, vaginal fluid, breast milk, saliva and tears. It is unable to survive or reproduce outside its living host but can effectively spread through sexual contact with an infected person. Highly active antiretroviral therapy became available in the late 1990s and changed the status of HIV from a fatal disease to a manageable chronic condition. However, cure is still not possible and highly active antiretroviral therapy remains expensive. Prevention remains vital. The proper (correct) and consistent (every time) use of condoms for sexual intercourse – vaginal, anal or oral – can greatly reduce a person's risk of acquiring or transmitting sexually transmitted infections, including HIV infection.

To be comprehensive, HIV programmes in prisons should include the following components:
- preventing new infections through, in particular: (1) reducing sexual transmission by improving life-skills (especially among younger prisoners), providing easy, anonymous access to condoms and lubricants, controlling sexually transmitted infections, notifying partners and implementing measures aimed at reducing sexual abuse and rape; (2) ensuring blood safety by testing transfused blood for HIV, reducing the number of nonvital blood transfusions and enrolling donors at lower risk; and (3) reducing transmission through sharing contaminated injecting equipment by implementing needle and syringe programmes, substitution therapy and peer-based education;
- mitigating HIV-related diseases by providing appropriate care, treatment (including highly active antiretroviral therapy) and support for HIV and related diseases;
- mitigating social impact by undertaking measures to counter HIV-related stigma and discrimination;
- conducting surveillance of HIV and AIDS; and
- providing easy access to voluntary HIV counselling and testing.

The United Nations Office on Drugs and Crime, UNAIDS and WHO (2006) recently released *HIV/AIDS prevention, care, treatment and support in prison settings: a framework for an effective national response.*

During the past decade, the treatment of people living with HIV has changed dramatically, with a resulting reduction of morbidity and mortality: a previously fatal disease has become a manageable chronic condition.

Although most of the people living with HIV in need worldwide still do not have access to this life-saving treatment, an initiative by WHO and UNAIDS to bring treatment to three million people in low-income countries by 2005 (the "3 by 5" Initiative), coupled with the unprecedented availability of funds from the Global Fund to Fight AIDS, Tuberculosis and Malaria, has resulted in rapid scale-up of antiretroviral therapy. This largely became possible because the treatment schemes were standardized and adapted to the context of resource-constrained settings. Using fixed-drug combinations solves several problems: daily tablet doses are significantly reduced, adherence improves and the risk of emergence of resistance is reduced, costs are lowered, logistics is easier and supervised treatment strategies are facilitated.

More recently, at the 2006 High Level Meeting on AIDS, the world committed to pursue all necessary efforts towards the goal of universal access to comprehensive prevention programmes, treatment, care and support by 2010.

Providing access to antiretroviral therapy for those in need in the context of prisons, particularly in resource-constrained settings, is a challenge, but it is necessary and feasible. Studies have documented that, when prisoners are provided care and access to antiretroviral therapy, they respond well. Adherence rates in prisons can be as high or higher than among people in the community, but the gains in health status made during the term of incarceration may be lost unless careful discharge planning and links to community care are undertaken.

As antiretroviral therapy is increasingly becoming available in low-income countries and countries in transition, ensuring that it also becomes available in the countries' prison systems will be critical. Ensuring continuity of care from the community to the prison and back to the community as well as continuity of care within the prison system is a fundamental component of successful efforts to scale up treatment.

Sustainable HIV treatment programmes in prisons, integrated into countries' general HIV treatment programmes or at least linked to them, are needed (Boxes 6.1 and 6.2).

Box 6.1 Strategies for treating HIV infection
- antiretroviral therapy to inhibit viral replication and induce immune reconstitution
- treating and preventing opportunistic infections and tumours
- preventing exposure to opportunistic infections

Box 6.2. WHO recommendations for staging HIV infection and disease
WHO recommends the following staging system for HIV infection and disease in adults and adolescents.
WHO clinical stage 1: asymptomatic
- no weight loss
- no symptoms or only persistent generalized lymphadenopathy
- performance scale 1: asymptomatic, normal activity

WHO clinical stage 2: mild disease
- weight loss 5–10%
- minor mucocutaneous manifestations, herpes zoster within past five years, recurrent upper respiratory tract infections (bacterial sinusitis or otitis)
- performance scale 2: symptomatic, normal activity

WHO clinical stage 3: moderate disease
- weight loss >10%
- unexplained chronic diarrhoea, or unexplained prolonged fever longer than one month, oral candidiasis (thrush), oral hairy leukoplakia, pulmonary tuberculosis within the past year, severe bacterial infections (such as pneumonia and pyomyositis)
- performance scale 3: bedridden <50% of the day during last month

WHO clinical stage 4: severe disease (AIDS)
- HIV wasting syndrome
- *Pneumocystis carinii* pneumonia, toxoplasmosis of the brain, cryptosporosis diarrhoea longer than one month, extrapulmonary cryptosporosis, cytomegalovirus disease other than liver, spleen or lymph node (retinitis), mucocutaneous or visceral herpes simplex virus infection, progressive multifocal leukoencephalopathy, any disseminated endemic mycosis, candidiasis of esophagus, trachea, bronchi, atypical *Mycobacterium tuberculosis* (disseminated or lungs), non-typhoid *Salmonella* septicaemia, extrapulmonary tuberculosis, lymphoma, Kaposi sarcoma, HIV encephalopathy

In its recommendations for initiating antiretroviral therapy among adults and adolescents, WHO distinguished between settings where CD4 testing is available and where they are not.

If CD4 testing is available, treatment starts at:
- WHO stage IV disease, irrespective of CD4 count;
- WHO stage III disease, consider (based on concomitant clinical conditions) using CD4 count <350 per mm3 to assist decision-making; and
- WHO stage I or II if CD4 count <200 per mm3.

If CD4 testing is not available, it is not recommended to treat asymptomatic adults with stage I. Treatment starts at:
- WHO stage IV disease, regardless of total lymphocyte count
- WHO stage III disease, regardless of total lymphocyte count
- WHO stage II or I disease with total lymphocyte count <1200 per mm3.

Many antiretroviral drugs are available – nucleoside and non-nucleoside reverse-transcriptase inhibitors and protease inhibitors (Box 6.3).

Box 6.3. WHO recommendations for antiretroviral therapy

First-line regimen
stavudine or zidovudine
+
lamivudine
+
nevirapine or efavirenz

Second-line regimen
tenofovir disoproxil fumarate or abacavir
+
didanosine
+
protease inhibitor: lopinavir with a low-dose ritonavir boost or saquinavir with a low-dose ritonavir boost

---

One serious problem of antiretroviral therapy is that any interruption of treatment can lead to resistance to at least some of the drugs used. Health staff should try to ensure compliance. In addition, other measures are needed to ensure that interruption of treatment does not occur. At the country level, (1) prison departments must have a place within the national HIV and AIDS coordinating committees, and prison issues need to be part of the agreed action framework for HIV and AIDS and country-level monitoring and evaluation system; (2) prison departments need to be involved in all aspects of scaling up treatment, from applications for funding (to ensure that funds are specifically earmarked for prisons), to developing, implementing and monitoring and evaluating plans for rolling out treatment; (3) the ministry responsible for health and the ministry responsible for the prison system should collaborate closely, recognizing that prison health is public health; alternatively, governments should assign responsibility for health care in prisons to the same ministries, departments and agencies that provide health care to people in the community; (4) guidelines should be developed specifying that people living with HIV are allowed to keep their medication upon them, or are to be provided with medication, upon arrest and incarceration and at any time they are transferred within the system or to court hearings. Police and correctional officers need to be educated about the importance of continuity of treatment. At the regional and local level, prisons should form partnerships with health clinics, hospitals and universities and nongovernmental organizations (including organizations of people living with HIV) to provide health care and other services for prisoners and to develop integrated rather than parallel care and treatment programmes.

People receiving antiretroviral therapy are regaining immune constitution, which may result in an inflammatory response for the first one to two months. Clinically this can manifest as fever, lymph node swelling, pulmonary and central nervous system involvement. People with latent tuberculosis infection can develop active tuberculosis. If active tuberculosis develops, antiretroviral therapy should not be stopped. Some special considerations apply to people with tuberculosis.
- Rifampicin interacts with nevirapine and protease inhibitors.
- The pill burden increases and adherence becomes more difficult to maintain.
- The first-line recommendation is: zidovudine or stavudine + lamivudine + efavirenz (600 or 800 mg/day), with zidovudine + lamivudine + abacavir being an alternative.
- The use of nevirapine is questioned due to likelihood of increased liver toxicity and poor efficacy.

Certain adverse effects are associated with use of antiretroviral drugs:
- mitochondrial toxicity with nucleotide reverse-transcriptase inhibitors;
- lactic acidosis, mitochondrial toxicity and lipodystrophy with nucleoside reverse-transcriptase inhibitors;
- skin rash and hepatitis with non-nucleoside reverse-transcriptase inhibitors; and
- lipodystrophy, hyperlipidaemia and hyperglycaemia with protease inhibitors.

Antiretroviral therapy requires clinical and laboratory assessments at baseline and regularly during therapy. Stage of HIV disease, concomitant conditions (tuberculosis and pregnancy), concomitant medication use (including traditional therapy), body weight and the patient's readiness for therapy are evaluated at baseline. While on therapy, signs and symptoms of potential drug toxicity, body weight, response to therapy and adherence are assessed and, when clinically indicated, depending on the antiretroviral drug regimen used, laboratory evaluation is performed.

Syphilis
Without treatment, the agent of syphilis, *Treponema pallidum*, persists in the body for life, leading to mutilation, nervous system disorders and death. Syphilis evolves in several phases, with symptoms varying with each phase.
- Primary syphilis: three weeks to three months after infection, painless wet ulcers (chancres) appear at the site of inoculation – genitals, anus, lips or mouth. The chancre lasts three to six weeks. The lymph nodes of the area may swell during the primary phase.
- Secondary syphilis: three to six weeks after the chancre, body rashes appear, often on the palms of the hands and the soles of the feet. Other symptoms include subfebrility, fatigue, sore throat, loss of hair in a patchy pattern (allopetia), weight loss, swollen lymph nodes, headache and muscle pains. The phase of secondary syphilis lasts for up to two years.

- Latent syphilis: this phase is characterized by the absence of any symptoms.
- Late syphilis: in untreated patients with syphilis, serious damage to the nervous system, heart, brain, and other viscera may occur and cause death.

Syphilis is spread through unprotected vaginal, anal and oral intercourse, through kissing, or from the mother to the fetus during pregnancy. It is most contagious in the early phases – the liquid that transudes from the chancre is highly infectious.

Diagnosis: blood samples are screened with serological tests. Dark-field microscopic examination of fluid from the chancre can confirm the diagnosis. Treatment: antibiotics are highly successful. *Treponema pallidum* is remarkably susceptible, and the disease is completely curable. However, the damage it can cause in the later phases is irreparable. Prevention: consistent use of condoms (for vaginal, anal and oral intercourse) reduces the risk of transmission.

Gonorrhoea

The agent of gonorrhoea is *Neisseria gonorrhoeae*, a bacterium that infects the urethra in men and women and the cervix, uterus and fallopian tubes in women. *Neisseria gonorrhoeae* can affect the mouth, throat, eyes and anus. Many men with gonorrhoea have no symptoms, but most develop symptoms two to five days after infection.

Symptoms: a burning sensation during urination and a white or greenish discharge from the penis. Occasionally men complain of painful or swollen testicles. Most women who are infected have no symptoms. When present, these symptoms are not highly specific for gonorrhoea: painful or burning urination, vaginal discharge or bleeding can indicate banal urinary tract infections. Rectal infection with Neisseria gonorrhoeae may cause no symptoms but can manifest itself through discharge, anal itching, soreness, bleeding or painful defecation.

Transmission: gonorrhoea is spread through contact with the penis, vagina, mouth or anus. Untreated gonorrhoea can cause serious complications. In women it can lead to infertility or extrauterine pregnancies through damage to the fallopian tubes. In men infertility occurs through epididymitis, an inflammatory condition of the testicles. Gonorrhoea can cause arthritis or sepsis, which is life-threatening.

Diagnosis: gonorrhoea can be diagnosed by Gram staining of a urethral sample and microscopy. Because gonorrhoea indicates high-risk sexual behaviour, tests for other sexually transmitted infections should be offered to all prisoners who are diagnosed with it.

Treatment: antibiotics can cure gonorrhoea, but drug-resistant strains of gonorrhoea are an increasing problem. It is important to ensure that the people with gonorrhoea are adherent and take a full course of medication. Even when infection is cured, the damage caused by the disease can be irreparable.

Prevention: using condoms reduces the risk of transmission of gonorrhoea. Inmates can be encouraged to stop having sex and to see a doctor whenever they have genital symptoms (such as discharge or burning at urination).

Trichomoniasis

Trichomoniasis is caused by monocellular protozoa.

Symptoms: women may notice foamy discharge with blood spots and itching in the vagina, painful, burning, frequent urinations, abdominal discomfort and painful intercourse. The symptoms develop 4 to 28 days after the contact. Men rarely have symptoms, and sometimes women do not have symptoms either.

Transmission: trichomoniasis is transmitted through vaginal intercourse. The diagnosis is made by microscopic examination of vaginal discharge or urethral specimens.

Treatment: trichomoniasis is treatable with imidazoles. Treating all partners simultaneously is important to prevent possible reinfection.

Prevention: proper use of condoms reduces the risk of infection. Limiting the number of sexual partners reduces the risk of encountering someone who has trichomoniasis.

Urinary tract infections

Urinary tract infections are caused by the ascension to the urethra and bladder of the rectal bacteria dislocated to the vagina or penis. This often occurs during sexual intercourse or sex play, but poor hygiene leading to contact of vagina or urethra with faeces can also result in urinary tract infections.

Urinary tract infections include cystitis; ureteritis (affecting the ureters) and urethritis (when the urethra is affected). Urinary tract infections that are left untreated may lead to kidney infection (pyelonephritis). Urinary tract infections are common among sexually active men and women. In general, women are more likely to be affected given the anatomy of a woman's urethra (shorter and closer to the anus). But in prisons, unprotected anal sex can expose male prisoners to an increased risk of urinary tract infections.

Symptoms of urinary tract infections include imperative, painful and sometimes involuntary urination, especially at night, lower abdominal pain or back pain, fever and blood and pus in the urine.

Diagnosis is usually based on clinical signs.

Antibiotics and symptomatic drugs are used for treatment.

To prevent urinary tract infections, inmates should use condoms during vaginal or anal intercourse, use lubricants, maintain the pubic area clean and dry, drink adequate liquids, urinate when they feel the urge and urinate immediately after intercourse.

Skin conditions

Scabies

The agent of scabies is an arachnoid that is most often sexually transmitted, but

in crowded prison environments inmates can also pass it to one another through casual contact, bedding and clothing. Itching is the most prominent symptom. It is particularly intense at night. Dirty-looking, curved lines are surrounded by small bumps and area of rashes. The favourite location is the thin skin of the penis, thighs, buttocks, around the navel and between the fingers. Usually, scabies does not present difficulties for clinical diagnosis. It is often self-diagnosed.
Scabies causes physical suffering and can be associated with serious bacterial infection.

For treatment, sulfur-containing prescriptions are applied neck-to-toe to all those who are affected or may have been exposed. All bedding, towels, and clothing that may have been exposed are autoclaved, boiled or dry-cleaned.

Pediculosis (head lice)
The agent of pediculosis is *Pediculus humanus capitis*, an insect parasiting the heads of people. Away from the host, the louse dies within two days. Pediculosis is a common condition in prisons, but reliable data on prevalence are rarely available. The lice are found in three forms: the nit, the nymph and the adult. Nits are the oval eggs of *Pediculus humanus capitis* that are attached to the hair. The nit hatches into a nymph. It takes about seven days for a nymph to mature, and in this interval nymphs feed on blood. The adult lice lay nits for about 30 days and feed on blood. The symptoms of pediculosis include the feeling that something is moving in the hair, itching, irascibility and occasionally infected sores resulting from scratching. The head lice are transmitted by contact with an infested person, wearing infested clothing and using infested combs, brushes, towels and bed linen. The diagnosis can be established by inspecting the hair for nits, nymphs or adults. In general, pediculosis only causes discomfort and inconvenience. Occasionally it can be complicated by secondary bacterial infections resulting from scratching. The treatment is with insecticides. Some kill lice, but not the unhatched nits, which requires a second treatment in 7–10 days. Most insecticides are safe if used correctly but can be dangerous if misused or overused. To prevent reinfestation and the further spread of pediculosis, all clothing and bed linens are washed with hot water or dry cleaned if they were in contact with the infested person in the last two days before the treatment. Alternatively, clothing can be stored in plastic bags and sealed for two weeks. Combs and brushes have to be washed with soap and hot water.

Infectious diseases of the digestive tract

Gastroenteritis
Gastroenteritis is an irritation and inflammation of the digestive tract. It is very prevalent both in the general population and in prisons. In most countries it is second only to the common cold in frequency of occurrence. The agents of gastroenteritis are very diverse: viruses, bacteria or parasites. Food poisoning, stress, alcohol or tobacco abuse, food allergies, inadequate diet, aspirin or corticoids can all cause gastroenteritis too, but viral and bacterial gastroenteritis can be easily transmitted.

Symptoms include loss of appetite, nausea, vomiting, diarrhoea, abdominal cramps, fever or chills, weakness and headache. Viral gastroenteritis usually lasts from several hours to several days. Bacterial or parasitic infections can last for more than one week and may require antibiotics for treatment. For a healthy person, the condition is as trivial as a common cold, but vomiting and diarrhoea can lead to dehydration and important metabolic disturbances. Elderly prisoners are at significant risk of shock from dehydration. Inflammatory damage to the intestinal mucosa can lead to diarrhoea that continues even after the initial infection is over. Diabetes mellitus and chronic liver or kidney problems put a person with gastroenteritis at additional risk for complications.

For treatment, prisoners should reduce their physical activity for the period of vomiting and diarrhoea; drink only clear liquids on day 1, until diarrhoea and vomiting stop; avoid solid foods and eat rice, crackers, soup and bread on day 2, and refrain from spicy fried food, dairy products, raw vegetables and fruits; drink 1.5–2.5 litres of liquid daily to balance the dehydration through diarrhoea and vomiting; and refrain from taking aspirin or ibuprofen. In severe cases a prison health worker can prescribe antiemetic and/or antispasmodic medication. This should be stopped as soon as the normal intestinal motility is restored. Prolonged diarrhoea can require testing and specific antibacterial treatment. Severe dehydration may occasionally require parenteral rehydration, and prisoners should seek health care if mucus or blood is found in stools, symptoms persist for more than 48 hours or if there is severe abdominal or rectal pain. Not every case of abdominal discomfort should be treated automatically as gastroenteritis. Surgical abdominal catastrophes can start with similar symptoms and have to be ruled out first.
Routine hygiene measures can effectively prevent infections that can cause gastroenteritis. Among these are: regularly cleaning and disinfecting toilets, washing hands after using the toilet, before eating or before preparing food; keeping raw meat and fish separate from cooked foods; and using individual towels.

Food poisoning
Food poisoning is an acute illness caused by ingesting food contaminated by bacteria, bacterial toxins, viruses, natural poisons (such as mushrooms) or chemicals. The most common causes are bacteria such as Staphylococcus aureus, Salmonella and pathogenic Escherichia coli. These bacteria are commonly found in the environment, but producing illness requires a large number of bacteria. Bacteria multiply best between 5°C and 65°C. Proper cooking and refrigeration greatly reduce the risk of food poisoning. Sometimes large groups of prisoners who ate the same food in prison or who shared homemade food brought by relatives can be infected at the same time. The symptoms of food poisoning can last for days and usually include abdominal cramps, diarrhoea, vomiting, nausea and fever. The onset is usually abrupt, and improvement occurs without any specific treatment. Severe cases can result in life-threatening nervous system, liver and kidney problems, occasionally leading to death. The measures that should be used to prevent food poisoning include: washing hands and utensils before and after handling raw foods to prevent cross-contamination, serving hot foods immediately or keeping them heated above 70°C to prevent bacteria from multiplying and heating canned foods for 5 to 10 minutes before tasting to destroy the toxins of botulism.

Reference
United Nations Office on Drugs and Crime, UNAIDS and WHO (2006). *HIV/AIDS prevention, care, treatment and support in prison settings: a framework for an effec-*

tive national response. Vienna, United Nations Office on Drugs and Crime (http://www.who.int/hiv/treatment/en/index.html, accessed 15 September 2006).

Further reading
University of Illinois, McKinley Health Center (2006). Health information handouts [web site]. Urbana, McKinley Health Center (http://www.mckinley.uiuc.edu/Handouts/list%20by%20topics.html, accessed 15 September 2006).
WHO (2000). *Tuberculosis control in prisons. A manual for programme managers.* Geneva, World Health Organization (http://www.who.int/docstore/gtb/publications/prisonsNTP/index.html, accessed 15 September 2006).

7. HIV infection and human rights in prisons - *Rick Lines*

Key points
- Efforts to reduce HIV-related stigma and discrimination must be part of effective and human rights-based policies and programmes on HIV infection in prisons.
- HIV-related stigma and discrimination often result in prison systems failing to meet their obligation to provide proper standards of health care.
- People in prison have a right to keep their personal medical information confidential. Ensuring this confidentiality is essential to providing effective and ethical care.
- Prisons must provide easy access to voluntary HIV testing, accompanied by pretest and post-test counselling.
- Mandatory HIV testing and forcible segregation of prisoners living with HIV are unethical and ineffective.
- Prison HIV and AIDS programmes benefit from collaboration with external nongovernmental organizations and health agencies, people living with HIV and prisoners themselves. This collaboration should be encouraged at all levels.

Setting the context: HIV-related stigma and discrimination in prisons
According to the Declaration of Commitment on HIV/AIDS, endorsed by the 189 countries represented at the United Nations General Assembly Special Session on HIV/AIDS in June 2001, "The vulnerable must be given priority in the response [to HIV/AIDS]". This statement is particularly relevant to addressing HIV and AIDS in prisons.

In many countries, the groups most vulnerable to or affected by HIV and AIDS are also groups at increased risk for criminalization and incarceration, as many of the same social and economic conditions that increase vulnerability to HIV and AIDS also increase vulnerability to imprisonment. As a result, in some countries the populations with the highest rates of HIV infection are also disproportionately represented within prisons. This has significant implications for prison health policy and must be addressed within a comprehensive response to HIV and AIDS in prisons.

Inside prisons, people living with HIV are often the most vulnerable and stigmatized segment of the prison population. Fear of HIV and AIDS often places HIV-positive prisoners at increased risk of social isolation, violence and human rights abuses from both prisoners and prison staff. In prisons, this fear is magnified by three factors:
- misinformation about routes of transmission (particularly the false belief that HIV can be transmitted via casual contact);
- the closed nature of the prison environment (particularly shared living, bathing and eating facilities, coupled with a culture of surveillance and monitoring); and
- stigma and discrimination against vulnerable groups (sex workers, people who use illegal drugs and homosexuals) within the prisoner population.

The fear of HIV and AIDS, and the social stigma of being known to be (or suspected of) living with HIV have negative effects on individuals and undermine the success of responses to HIV and AIDS. For example, fear of potential discrimination can deter prisoners from accessing voluntary HIV testing. It can also discourage prisoners living with HIV from seeking health care services. Combating stigma and discrimination related to HIV and AIDS in prisons is therefore important to protecting the rights of prisoners living with HIV and to increasing the effectiveness of HIV and AIDS services.

As mentioned in chapter 2, declarations and guidelines from numerous international bodies and organizations support the principle that people in prison have a right to be provided with a standard of health care equivalent to that available in the community and should not be subjected to inadequate health care simply because of their status as prisoners. International instruments supporting this "principle of equivalence" include the United Nations Basic Principles for the Treatment of Prisoners,[8] the WHO *Guidelines on HIV infection and AIDS in prisons*[9] *and the United Nations International Guidelines on HIV/AIDS and Human Rights*,[10] among others. UNAIDS has also supported this principle in testimony before the United Nations Commission on Human Rights.[11] Indeed, it can be argued that governments owe a higher standard of care to people in detention, given the extreme health problems found among prison populations worldwide and the obligations of a state under international law to protect the lives and well-being of people it holds in custody (Lines, 2006).

The principle of equivalence is fundamental to the promotion of human rights and proper health care standards within prisons. Although HIV-related stigma and discrimination create barriers to achieving this standard, prison systems can and must take proactive steps in many key areas to ensure that proper standards of HIV and AIDS care, based on human rights norms and medical ethics, are implemented.

A core element in developing effective health care and social responses to HIV/AIDS in prisons is therefore creating a framework – in policy, legislation, education programmes and staff training – that counters stigma and discrimination and false information about HIV and AIDS. In addition, the existence and negative impact of HIV-related stigma and discrimination must be recognized and addressed in developing effective and human rights–based responses to HIV and AIDS in prisons.

Confidentiality in prison
Prisons are closed societies in which security and surveillance are central parts of everyday life. Within this environment, absolute confidentiality may be impossible

[8] World Medical Association Declaration on Hunger Strikers Adopted by the 43rd World Medical Assembly Malta, November 1991 and revised by the WMA General Assembly, Pilanesberg, South Africa, October 2006
[9] World Medical Association Declaration on Hunger Strikers Adopted by the 43rd World Medical Assembly Malta, November 1991 and revised by the WMA General Assembly, Pilanesberg, South Africa, October 2006
[10] World Medical Association Declaration on Hunger Strikers Adopted by the 43rd World Medical Assembly Malta, November 1991 and revised by the WMA General Assembly, Pilanesberg, South Africa, October 2006
[11] World Medical Association Declaration on Hunger Strikers Adopted by the 43rd World Medical Assembly Malta, November 1991 and revised by the WMA General Assembly, Pilanesberg, South Africa, October 2006

to achieve. Yet despite the challenges, policies and practices that maximize confidentiality – both in appearance and in fact – must be implemented to ensure an effective and rights-based response to HIV and AIDS.

Prisoners living with HIV routinely face social isolation, discrimination and even violence as a result of their HIV status. This stigma and discrimination causes stress and fear for prisoners living with HIV, and also discourage others from seeking testing and/or accessing treatment. For this reason, the confidentiality of HIV status is of primary importance to many prisoners living with HIV.

Within the prison setting, confidentiality may be broken in both deliberate and subtle ways.

For example, in many countries a lack of education and training among prison staff results in the mistaken belief that a prisoner's HIV status is a workplace safety issue. In these conditions, prison guards often believe they have the right to know which prisoners are living with HIV because they falsely believe that such information will protect them from workplace exposure to HIV. If such misinformation is not challenged, it can promote an environment in which staff commonly, or even routinely, breach confidentiality. This undermines staff safety by promoting a false understanding of workplace "risk" and "safety". It also violates the right to the medical confidentiality of prisoners and can encourage a working atmosphere in which members of health care staff are pressured to disclose medical information to non-medical staff, such as prison officers and prison officials.

Confidentiality may also be undermined by other prisoners who, like prison officers, mistakenly believe that identifying people living with HIV will protect them from HIV infection. Misinformation about HIV and AIDS can create fears about the risk of HIV transmission via shared living spaces, shared bathing areas, shared food, etc. Such attitudes can undermine the effectiveness of HIV prevention initiatives among prisoners by creating an atmosphere in which identifying prisoners living with HIV – rather than reducing high-risk behaviour – is considered the most effective manner to protect oneself against HIV infection. These attitudes also sustain an atmosphere of discrimination, and potential violence, against people living with HIV.

Within prisons, confidentiality may also be compromised in more subtle, less deliberate, ways. For example, prisoners known to be living with HIV may have special marks or labels placed on their prison files, medical files or prison cells. Institutional practices for providing health care appointments, delivering HIV test results and dispensing medication may also differ for prisoners living with HIV than for HIV-negative prisoners, a fact that other prisoners and prison staff will notice. Prison officers may choose to follow certain routines with prisoners known (or suspected of) living with HIV that they do not follow with all prisoners, such as wearing latex gloves. All these actions potentially disclose a person's HIV status.

Prison staff, who deliberately breach the duty of confidentiality owed to prisoners, breach prisoners' right to privacy (Betteridge, 2004). Ensuring the privacy of medical information is particularly crucial to the credibility of prison health care staff. Unless prisoners are able to trust that their medical information is secure, they will be less likely to access health care services for HIV testing and treatment. They will also be more likely to shy away from counselling and education on HIV prevention.

Despite the inherent challenges, international standards established by WHO (1993), the World Medical Association (2004) and others state that prisoners have a right to have their medical information treated with the same level of confidentiality as patients outside prisons. The WHO (1993) *Guidelines on HIV infection and AIDS in prisons* are particularly clear on this and state that "information on the health status and medical treatment of prisoners is confidential" and can only be disclosed by medical staff with the prisoner's consent or where "warranted to ensure the safety and well-being of prisoners and staff, applying to the disclosure the same principles as generally applied in the community".

Prison systems have an obligation to ensure that breaches of confidentiality are not tolerated and to implement specific policies on confidentiality, train staff on the purpose and use of these policies and impose sanctions on staff who violate these policies.

HIV testing and pretest and post-test counselling

The principle of equivalence mandates that the quality and scope of health care services in prisons meet the standards of that provided in the outside community. This principle should also apply to HIV testing.

The WHO (1993) *Guidelines on HIV infection and AIDS in prisons* state the following:

Voluntary testing for HIV infection should be available in prisons when available in the community, together with adequate pretest and post-test counselling. Voluntary testing should only be carried out with the informed consent of the prisoner. Support should be available when prisoners are notified of test results and in the period following.

However, in many countries providing HIV testing services in prisons does not meet the standard in the wider community. Some prison systems provide no access – or limited access – to HIV testing. In prison systems where HIV testing is available, testing sometimes takes places without proper pretest and post-test counselling or without adequate support for prisoners who receive a positive test result. Prisoners are often very concerned about confidentiality, and this may discourage them from participating in testing.

Addressing these common problems requires that testing protocols be developed that maximize prisoner confidence in the process and in the privacy of their test results.

WHO advocates that all HIV testing – including testing in prisons – follow the principle known as the three C's. According to these principles (UNAIDS and WHO, 2004), HIV testing must be:
- confidential
- accompanied by counselling
- only be conducted with informed consent (consent that it is both informed and voluntary).

A person providing informed consent must be provided information about (UNAIDS and WHO, 2004):
- the benefits of testing for the individual and for the community;
- the person's right to refuse testing;
- the services that will be offered following the test result; and
- if the person tests positive, the importance of anticipating the need to inform anyone at ongoing risk who would otherwise not suspect they were being exposed to HIV infection.

This applies to all forms of HIV testing, including rapid HIV tests.
HIV testing must include counselling both before the test and upon communicating the results. According to WHO (Perriens et al., 2000):

Counselling is important to prepare clients to come to terms with their HIV status: this includes dealing with fear, guilt, stigma, discrimination, care for a chronic condition, the possibility of early death, and to give them an understanding of what they can and should do about HIV infection, should they be HIV-infected. It is also important in helping people devise or strengthen ways of staying HIV negative, if they test HIV negative.

Pretest counselling should assess the prisoner's risk of HIV infection and the window period (the last time the person engaged in unsafe behaviour) and should provide information on HIV infection, strategies to avoid or reduce the risk of HIV infection and the advantages and disadvantages of testing. Post-test counselling should include communicating the test result, assessing the prisoner's understanding of the result, assessing the need for follow-up care and highlighting the importance of risk-reducing behaviour regardless of the test result (Bollini, 2001).

Prison health care staff should be properly trained on the importance of pretest and post-test counselling and provided the resources to implement counselling in all cases. Maximizing participation in voluntary HIV testing requires maintaining confidentiality at all stages of the process – pretest counselling, the testing itself, communication of test results to the prisoner and post-test counselling and any follow-up support or care.

Coercive approaches are counterproductive
It has generally been accepted that coercive and discriminatory approaches to HIV are not in the best interests of the individual or of society as a whole. If people living with HIV – or at risk of HIV infection – fear discrimination or a lack of medical confidentiality, they are less likely to come forward for voluntary testing or to access counselling and education on HIV prevention measures (Bollini, 2001).

Nevertheless, some prison systems tend to opt for the types of coercive and discriminatory approaches that have been largely rejected outside prisons. Mandatory HIV testing and forcible isolation of people living with HIV are two such coercive policies that are still practised – either formally or informally – in many prisons of the world.

Mandatory HIV testing

Since the HIV epidemic began, the issue of mandatory HIV testing of prisoners has been widely debated. In some prison systems, mandatory HIV testing (testing without the consent of the prisoner) remains standard practice. In some cases, all incoming prisoners are subjected to non-consensual testing. In others, mandatory testing is targeted at prisoners identified as being at "high risk".

Some prison authorities have supported mandatory HIV testing as a strategy for preventing HIV transmission, based on the mistaken belief that identifying people known to be infected with HIV will help prevent transmission to others. In other cases, mandatory HIV testing has been proposed as a strategy to improve health care by identifying prisoners living with HIV and providing early referral to health services.

However, mandatory HIV testing has no place in an effective and rights-based HIV and AIDS strategy. Mandatory HIV testing is not considered an appropriate response to HIV infection in the community outside prison, and it is therefore equally inappropriate in prisons. As Betteridge (2004) explained, "HIV antibody testing performed without consent potentially infringes the right to security of the person, the right not to be subjected to torture or to cruel, inhuman or degrading treatment or punishment, and the right to privacy." Many of the prison systems that introduced a policy of mandatory testing early on later abandoned it, acknowledging that it is both costly and inefficient (Betteridge, 2004).

In addition to the human rights and ethical problems inherent in using mandatory HIV testing, the practice is not supported on medical or preventive grounds. The nature of HIV antibody testing means that a prison will never be able to accurately identify all prisoners infected with HIV. The window period inherent in the testing technology – which means that it may take up to 14 weeks and perhaps longer for a person infected with HIV to develop HIV antibodies in a sufficient concentration to trigger a positive test result – means that false-negative test results are unavoidable.

The *Guidelines on HIV infection and AIDS in prisons* (WHO, 1993) clearly oppose the use of mandatory HIV testing, stating that mandatory HIV testing of prisoners is "unethical and ineffective, and should be prohibited".

Forced segregation of prisoners living with HIV

Like mandatory HIV testing, the forced segregation or isolation of people living with HIV has been widely debated in prison systems over the years. In some cases, segregation of prisoners living with HIV has been supported as an HIV prevention strategy, on the mistaken belief that isolating prisoners living with HIV would prevent further HIV transmission in the prison. In other cases, segregation has been supported on medical grounds, on the basis that better care can be provided to prisoners living with HIV housed together in a special living unit. Yet whatever the rationale, forced segregation is an inappropriate and unethical response to HIV and AIDS in prisons.

Because HIV cannot be transmitted via casual contact (as can active tuberculosis, for example – see chapter 8 for a discussion of the segregation of people with tuberculosis), the forced isolation of people living with HIV serves no credible preventive purpose. However, forced segregation can promote several negative outcomes that would undermine efforts to prevent HIV transmission and to care for prisoners living with HIV. It also has implications for the rights of people living with HIV.

Forced segregation can be a significant deterrent to the uptake of voluntary HIV testing. If prisoners know or fear that they will be segregated if found to be HIV-positive, many will choose not to test rather than test and risk segregation. In the same way, forced segregation can act as a deterrent to accessing health care. Prisoners living with HIV may choose not to identify themselves to health care staff if doing so means that they will be segregated from their friends and peers. Mandatory segregation policies can therefore result in deterring prisoners living with HIV from accessing necessary health care.

Like mandatory testing, forced segregation also increases and entrenches HIV-related stigma and discrimination among prisoners and prison staff by creating the impression that prisoners living with HIV are a "danger". This increases the vulnerability of people living with HIV to human rights abuses from prisoners and prison staff.

Forced segregation can also undermine broader HIV prevention initiatives among prisoners and staff by creating the unrealistic and dangerous assumption that all prisoners living with HIV are segregated, and that therefore there is "no HIV" in the general prison population. This can result in increased risk behaviour in prisons by leading other prisoners to believe they need not practise safer sex or safer needle use and prison staff to believe they need not take universal precautions.

The *Guidelines on HIV infection and AIDS in prisons* (WHO, 1993) oppose forced segregation or isolation, stating, "Since segregation, isolation and restrictions on occupational activities, sports and recreation are not considered useful or relevant in the case of HIV-infected people in the community, the same attitude should be adopted towards HIV-infected prisoners."

Segregation or isolation should only be considered when it is required for the well-being of a prisoner living with HIV and the prisoner requests it, such as when the prisoner's health may be jeopardized by viruses or opportunistic infections transmitted by others in the prison population or when other means such as education and discipline of fellow prisoners have failed to protect the prisoner living with HIV from violence. Segregation or isolation may also be necessary when a prisoner living with HIV is violent or predatory. However, decisions about the segregation of prisoners living with HIV in these cases should follow the same criteria as decisions about the segregation of any other prisoner. If prisoners are violent or predatory, their actions may justify isolation or other disciplinary measures regardless of their HIV status.

Finally, prisoners living with HIV should not be excluded from any educational, job or vocational programme, and in particular from working in kitchens and infirmaries, by reason of their HIV status alone.

Addressing concerns about trust and confidentiality: working with nongovernmental organizations, people living with HIV, peers and professionals outside the prison system

One of the most effective strategies for addressing the confidentiality concerns that create barriers to effective HIV and AIDS programmes is to collaborate with individuals and groups from outside the prison service. Staff from agencies outside the prison (nongovernmental organizations, community-based organizations and community health clinics) can make a valuable contribution to developing and delivering HIV and AIDS initiatives in prisons, including HIV prevention programmes, HIV testing services and emotional support and counselling.

Experience with HIV and AIDS services in many prison systems has shown that prisoners can develop more trust with staff from nongovernmental organizations and other professionals from outside the prison than they can with staff who are part of the prison hierarchy. This is because workers from outside the prison are often considered more independent – and therefore more confidential – than are prison employees, and as a result prisoners may be more willing to openly discuss subjects such as risk behaviour and HIV status.

Several prison systems have developed partnerships with voluntary HIV testing clinics from the local community and have arranged for the staff from these clinics to come into the prisons on an ongoing basis to provide HIV testing services to prisoners. Because the clinic staff members are not part of the prison system, prisoners may be more willing to opt for voluntary testing, as they have greater trust that their results will not be disclosed to the prison staff. Such partnerships have also benefited the prison itself, as they have provided additional support and resources for often overburdened prison health care units.

Similar collaborative arrangements have been developed in some countries to provide HIV prevention education programmes and counselling for prisoners living with HIV. Again, the perceived independence of outside groups can be an advantage in encouraging prisoners to discuss delicate personal issues such as sexuality and drug use. The active involvement of agencies from outside the prison can also increase the support available to prisoners upon their release and thereby provide assistance in community reintegration and continuity of care and services.

The *Guidelines on HIV infection and AIDS in prisons* (WHO, 1993) recommend the following.

Cooperation with relevant nongovernmental and private organizations, such as those with expertise in AIDS prevention, counselling and social support, should be encouraged. HIV-infected prisoners should have access to voluntary agencies and other sources of advice and help.

Collaboration with people living with HIV, and with prisoners themselves in peer-based initiatives, can also play an important role in boosting the credibility and effectiveness of HIV and AIDS programmes in prisons.

Involving people living with HIV (or at risk of contracting HIV) in designing and implementing HIV and AIDS programmes is an important part of an effective response to HIV and AIDS, as recognized by the Declaration of Commitment on HIV/AIDS (UNAIDS, 2001). The development of peer support (UNAIDS, 1999), peer education and peer self-help groups – in which members of the target population themselves are trained to act as supporters and educators for their own peer group – can also make a valuable contribution to effective HIV and AIDS services.

However, prison officials have too often neglected – or actively discouraged – such approaches. For example, people living with HIV from outside the prisons – particularly those who currently use drugs or have done so in the past or those who have past criminal convictions – may not be allowed into prisons as part of programmes. Prison staff often see prisoners themselves as a threat to security, especially prisoners who use drugs or those seen as "leaders" within the prison population, and exclude them from participating in developing and delivering peer-based HIV and AIDS programmes. In order to maximize the diversity and effectiveness of HIV and AIDS services in prisons, such barriers should be overcome and full participation encouraged by these groups.

Compassionate or early release
Prisoners who enter the later stages of chronic or terminal illnesses – including but not limited to HIV and AIDS – require specialized end-of-life care. Prisons – even in high-income countries – are ill equipped to provide such care.

End-of-life care is unique and demanding, and prison staff often lack the necessary training and resources. The prison environment itself – with its security-focused architecture and routines, lack of comfort and privacy, barriers to access for family and friends – is also generally not conducive to compassionate and responsive end-of-life care. Proper end-of-life care – particularly in the context of HIV and AIDS – often involves providing large doses of pain management medication, which may conflict with the "drug-free" ethos of the prison system.

For these reasons, many prison systems have introduced compassionate release programmes to allow terminally ill prisoners to be released from prison earlier in their sentence. Such early-release programmes fulfil a compassionate role but also recognize that the life expectancy of terminally ill prisoners may be lengthened as a result of receiving care in the community.

The Guidelines on HIV infection and AIDS in prisons (WHO, 1993) recommend the compassionate release of terminally ill prisoners.

If compatible with considerations of security and judicial procedures, prisoners with advanced AIDS should be granted compassionate early release, as far as possible, in order to facilitate contact with their families and friends and to allow them to face death with dignity and in freedom.

Conclusion
More than two decades of experience in addressing HIV and AIDS in prisons internationally has demonstrated the value of developing policies and programmes

that are consistent with human rights standards. Indeed, protecting and fulfilling human rights, including countering the negative effects of HIV-related stigma and discrimination, should be seen as a key element in developing effective and ethical responses to HIV and AIDS in prison.

References

Betteridge G (2004). *Prisoners' health & human rights in the HIV/AIDS epidemic – background paper.* Montreal, Canadian HIV/AIDS Legal Network.

Bollini P, ed. (2001). *HIV in prisons: a reader with particular relevance to the Newly Independent States.* Copenhagen, WHO Regional Office for Europe (http://www.euro.who.int/document/e77016.pdf, accessed 15 September 2006).

Lines R (2006). From equivalence of standards to equivalence objectives: the entitlement of prisoners to health standards higher than those outside prisons. *International Journal of Prisoner Health*, 2:269–280.

Office of the United Nations High Commissioner for Human Rights and UNAIDS (1997). *International Guidelines on HIV/AIDS and Human Rights.* U.N.C.H.R. res. 1997/33, U.N. Doc. E/CN.4/1997/150 (1997).

Office of the United Nations High Commissioner for Human Rights and UNAIDS (2006). *International guidelines on HIV/AIDS and human rights.* Consolidated version. Geneva, Office of the United Nations High Commissioner for Human Rights.

Perriens J et al. (2000). *Key elements in HIV/AIDS care and support: a working document.* Geneva, World Health Organization and UNAIDS.

UNAIDS (1997). Statement on HIV/AIDS in prisons to the United Nations Commission on Human Rights at its Fifty-second Session, April 1996. In: *UNAIDS, prison and AIDS: UNAIDS point of view.* Geneva, UNAIDS.

UNAIDS (1999). *Peer education and HIV/AIDS: concepts, uses and challenges.* Geneva, UNAIDS (http://data.unaids.org/Publications/IRC-pub01/JC291-PeerEduc_en.pdf, accessed 15 September 2006).

UNAIDS (2001). Belarus – involving young people, nongovernmental organizations and the target population in preventing HIV/AIDS. In: *Drug abuse and HIV/AIDS: lessons learned. Case studies booklet. Central and eastern Europe and the central Asian states.* Geneva, UNAIDS.

UNAIDS and WHO (2004). *UNAIDS/WHO policy statement on HIV testing, June 2004.* Geneva, UNAIDS and WHO (http://www.who.int/hiv/pub/vct/statement/en/index.html, accessed 15 September 2006).

United Nations (1990). *Basic Principles for the Treatment of Prisoners. Adopted and proclaimed by General Assembly resolution 45/111 of 14 December 1990.* New York, United Nations.

WHO (1993). *Guidelines on HIV infection and AIDS in prisons.* Geneva, World Health Organization, 1993 (http://whqlibdoc.who.int/hq/1993/WHO_GPA_DIR_93.3.pdf, accessed 15 September 1006).

World Medical Association (2000). *Declaration of Edinburgh on Prison Conditions and the Spread of Tuberculosis and Other Communicable Diseases.* Helsinki, World Medical Association.

Further reading

Lines R (1997–1998). The case against segregation in "specialized" care units. *Canadian HIV/AIDS Policy & Law Newsletter*, 3(4) and 4(1):30–35.

Lines R (2002). *Pros & cons: a guide to creating successful community-based*

HIV/AIDS programs for prisoners. Toronto, Prisoners' HIV/AIDS Support Action Network.

UNAIDS (2001). *Drug abuse and HIV/AIDS: lessons learned. Case studies booklet. Central and eastern Europe and the central Asian states. Geneva,* UNAIDS.

United Nations Office on Drugs and Crime, World Health Organization and UNAIDS (2006). *HIV/AIDS prevention, care, treatment and support in prison settings: a framework for an effective national response.* New York: United Nations Office on Drugs and Crime, World Health Organization and UNAIDS.

16. Tuberculosis control in prisons - *Jaap Veen*

Key points
- Tuberculosis is a public health problem in many countries of the WHO European Region, more widespread in eastern than in western countries.
- Due to overcrowding and poor nutrition, tuberculosis rates in many prisons are 10 to 100 times higher than in the community outside prisons.
- Since many prisoners come from marginalized populations, in which both tuberculosis and injecting drug use are most prevalent, the occurrence of dual infection with tuberculosis and HIV in prison inmates is not rare.
- There are three strategies for tuberculosis case-finding: 1) self-referral; 2) screening at entry to the prison; and 3) active case-finding among prisoners.
- The best strategy for preventing tuberculosis in correctional facilities is early diagnosis combined with effective treatment.
- Proper treatment reduces coughing in two to three weeks. If the bacilli are sensitive to the drugs used, most will be killed within a month. Treatment is needed for a minimum of six months and often longer.
- Simple cough hygiene is very effective. Covering mouth and nose when coughing or sneezing significantly reduces the number of bacilli in the air.
- Ventilation is very effective and can easily be obtained by opening windows. Ultraviolet irradiation (sunlight) is also effective, but only when sunlight can reach the bacilli. Artificial ultraviolet devices can be used under specific conditions.
- People with infectious tuberculosis should be kept separate from people with non-infectious tuberculosis. Isolation should not be equated with punishment or solitary confinement.
- It is important that people with tuberculosis adhere to regular drug intake.
- Prison tuberculosis control programmes should have the same standards as the tuberculosis programmes in the general community and use the same guidelines and protocols.
- Prison staff and prisoners should receive health education. Overcrowding, lack of ventilation, heavy smoking and lack of general hygiene contribute to the transmission of tuberculosis.
- Prison administration should regularly evaluate the efficacy of methods to identify the infectious people and the strategies to contain tuberculosis. tuberculosis is not an unavoidable consequence of incarceration and can be controlled by applying DOTS-based programmes and improving prison conditions.
- Effective tuberculosis control in prison protects prisoners, staff, visitors and the community at large.

Introduction
Prisons are extremely high-risk environments for infectious diseases because of overcrowding, poor nutrition, limited access to health care, continued drug use and unsafe injecting practices, unprotected sex and tattooing. A recent review (Niveau, 2006) identified the three main risk factors for infectious diseases in correctional facilities as being proximity, high-risk sexual behaviour and injecting drug use.
The review suggested that preventive measures for four diseases be given priority: tuberculosis, HIV, hepatitis and sexually transmitted infections. This chapter deals with tuberculosis.

What is tuberculosis?
Tuberculosis is a public health problem in many countries of the WHO European Region. In western European countries, tuberculosis is mainly concentrated in people born in other countries, homeless people, people with drug dependence and prisoners. Eastern European countries still have a high general burden of tuberculosis, compounded by the growing HIV epidemic (Drobniewski, 2005), and prisons in eastern Europe have often been cited as reservoirs of tuberculosis.

Transmission and natural progress
Tuberculosis is an infectious disease caused by a bacillus named *Mycobacterium tuberculosis*. Transmission occurs by airborne droplets, produced by coughing or sneezing, that are subsequently inhaled by contact people. The risk of inhalation increases when more coughing people are kept in a small, unventilated room. In general, about 30% of contacts that inhale bacilli become infected. But in prisons with overcrowding and poor nutrition, twice as many contacts or more could become infected. Smoking seems to aggravate the risk of becoming infected.

Depending on the infected person's immune system, infection may result in disease. Immunity is determined by many factors, both physical and mental. tuberculosis rates in prisons are 10 to 100 times higher than in the community outside prisons. tuberculosis-infected people who are also living with HIV are more than 100 times more likely to develop active tuberculosis than people who are not HIV infected.

When no treatment is available, at least half of those with tuberculosis disease die within two years; some may heal spontaneously and others become chronic cases that continue to transmit the disease.

Clinical patterns
The disease starts in the lungs after inhalation and has its most frequent manifestation in the lungs: pulmonary tuberculosis. The predominant feature of tuberculosis is the formation of abscesses. As long as these abscesses are contained, there is no risk of transmission (closed tuberculosis). But if these abscesses break through into the airways, the infectious content will be coughed up (open tuberculosis). Abscesses contain billions of bacilli. People with open tuberculosis are highly infectious. About 50–60% of people with tuberculosis eventually become infectious.

The bloodstream can carry bacilli to other parts of the body, where they may cause serious illness, such as meningitis or septicaemia. Almost all organs can be affected. This occurs in about 15–20% of people with tuberculosis.

The risk of becoming infected and subsequently developing tuberculosis disease depends on a number of risk factors. In prison these risk factors reinforce each other. The longer a prisoner is incarcerated the higher becomes the risk of developing tuberculosis (Bellin, 1993).

Diagnosis
Tuberculosis infection can be detected by a tuberculin skin test. But many factors influence the reliability of this test, and the test is only used in specific circumstances.

To demonstrate the presence of tuberculosis disease, a chest X-ray helps in identifying whether any abnormality is present, but it cannot be decisive for the diagnosis. Only bacteriological examination can provide proof of the existence of tuberculosis. Microscopic examination of sputum may result in a diagnosis on the same day. To confirm the diagnosis, sputum must be cultured. Depending on the technique used, growth becomes visible after 2–8 weeks. Modern molecular techniques that can confirm the diagnosis more rapidly have become available, but they are costly and not reliable enough under routine conditions.

Treatment

Five first-line drugs are available for normal tuberculosis treatment. A combination of these drugs has to be taken regularly to prevent the development of resistance. Each drug dose includes several tablets. To prevent mistakes, health care staff should supervise the administration of each dose (direct observed therapy (DOT)). The usual treatment duration is 6–8 months.

Because many tablets have to be taken, ideally under direct observation, and because of the long duration of treatment, achieving treatment success in prisons is quite complicated.

Epidemiology

Information on the number of prisoners, prisoners with tuberculosis and tuberculosis infection control policies within correctional systems is scarce. In 2002, WHO estimated the total prison population of the WHO European Region at 2.1 million, with more than 10.5 million people passing through the penitentiary system every year.

A survey (Aerts et al., 2006) found that the mean tuberculosis notification rate per 100 000 prisoners in Europe in 2003 was 1516, ranging from 0 in Cyprus, Malta and Norway to 3944 in Azerbaijan and 17 808 in Kazakhstan. Eastern European countries accounted for 93% of prisoners with tuberculosis in this survey. Based on these figures, an estimated 32 000 prisoners had tuberculosis in prisons in Europe in 2003, of which 30 000 were in countries of the former Soviet Union.

Multidrug-resistant tuberculosis

A very serious form of tuberculosis that is resistant to the usual anti-tuberculosis drugs has developed in recent years. Multidrug-resistant tuberculosis is especially prevalent in prisons in eastern Europe, where 30–50% of prisoners with tuberculosis probably have multidrug-resistant tuberculosis. Second-line drugs, in large quantities and for a very long duration (18 to 24 months), must be administered to people with multidrug-resistant tuberculosis. These drugs are weak, are very expensive, create many adverse effects and are not always in sufficient supply on the world market.

An outbreak of multidrug-resistant tuberculosis in New York State prisons demonstrated how failing to control the disease within prisons affected the health of the community at large.

Tuberculosis/HIV

HIV infection is the largest individual risk factor for developing tuberculosis. Since the emergence of the HIV and AIDS epidemic, dual tuberculosis/HIV epidemics have emerged in all regions of the world. The HIV epidemic drives the global tuberculosis epidemic.

As many prisoners come from marginalized populations in which both tuberculosis and injecting drug use are not uncommon, the occurrence of dual infection with tuberculosis and HIV in prison inmates is not rare. Spain had very high rates of HIV infection among injecting drug users before it introduced and expanded effective HIV prevention measures such as needle and syringe programmes and substitution therapy. A cohort study in a prison in which a tuberculosis programme was run from 1991 to 1999 (Martin et al., 2001) showed that 10% of the 1050 prisoners studied were coinfected with HIV and tuberculosis. HIV infection rates have increased rapidly in countries of the former Soviet Union since the mid- to late 1990s, and tuberculosis/HIV is also increasing there in prisons. The continuous ongoing transmission of tuberculosis, including multidrug-resistant tuberculosis, will be aggravated by an increasing number of prisoners whose immune system is seriously compromised by HIV infection.

What can be done to reduce the risk of transmission of tuberculosis?
Prisons are not closed environments, as inmates are constantly in contact with the outside world through visitors and prison staff. In addition, inmates enter, leave and re-enter prisons regularly. In several countries, a strong association between tuberculosis prevalence in correctional facilities and in the community outside prisons has been reported. Interventions to reduce the risk of transmission of tuberculosis in prisons are therefore not only important for prisoners and prison staff but provide a direct public service to the community outside the walls of the correctional institutions.

Interventions to interrupt the cycle of transmission can be directed at two levels: 1) preventing transmission of tuberculosis from people with infectious tuberculosis to their contacts, and 2) preventing the disease from developing once any contacts have become infected (Fig. 8.1).

Fig. 8.1. The cycle of tuberculosis transmission
Change infection

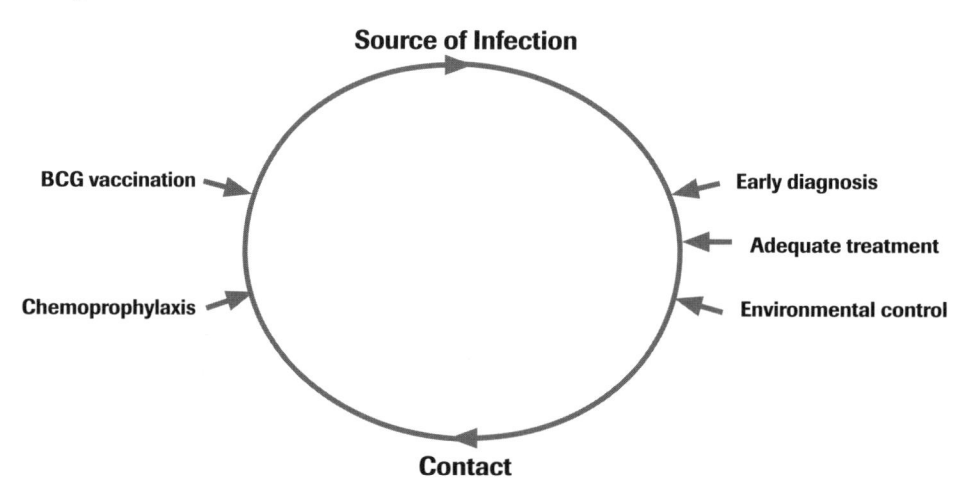

To prevent transmission, early case detection, immediate and adequate treatment and infection control interventions are needed. To prevent infected contacts from developing active disease, vaccination and preventive chemotherapy may be considered.

There are three strategies for case-finding: 1) through self-referral; 2) through screening at entry to the prison; and 3) active case-finding among prisoners.

Self-referral
Patients with respiratory (or other) symptoms of tuberculosis should seek and find health care. For case-finding to be effective, patients must be aware that the symptoms they experience may be symptoms of tuberculosis and that tuberculosis can be treated, must be willing to seek diagnosis and treatment and must be able to access tuberculosis care (WHO, 2000). Educating everyone in prison about tuberculosis is therefore important.

However, case-finding through self-referral may have limited success in prisons. Some inmates may be afraid to come forward, fearing the repercussions of a diagnosis of tuberculosis, such as the stigma tuberculosis brings with it, a transfer to another facility or a delay in their release. Sometimes inmates may not be allowed to seek care because of their place in the internal hierarchy among the prisoners.

Screening for tuberculosis at entry
The revised European Prison Rules (Committee of Ministers of the Council of Europe, 2006) state that prisoners are entitled to a medical examination at the point of first admission (§42) and that prison authorities have to safeguard the health of all prisoners (§39). Medical screening at entry into the prison system is essential, as many prisoners come from communities with high tuberculosis prevalence. Prisoners should not enter the body of the prison population until it has been verified that they do not have infectious tuberculosis.

Active case-finding
Periodically and systematically screening the entire prison population can substantially influence the transmission of tuberculosis in prisons. How frequently such screening should be undertaken depends on several factors, including the prevalence of the disease and the availability of financial and human resources. Where the prevalence is high (such as in eastern European prisons), the entire prison population needs to be screened every six months. The methods for case-finding are 1) tuberculin skin testing; 2) radiography; and 3) questionnaires.

Tuberculin skin testing, as stated earlier, is a weak tool for detecting tuberculosis infection in high-prevalence settings and is rarely used in prisons. Radiography is relatively easy to organize, but the disadvantage is the high cost involved in capital investment, operating costs and maintenance. It also requires expertise in reading films. Questionnaires to be filled in by the prisoners are inexpensive but can be subject to great bias. They may identify a large proportion of people who need diagnostic procedures.

Whatever screening method is used, everyone suspected of having tuberculosis should have their sputum examined.

Adequate treatment

Another way of preventing transmission is to start adequate treatment as soon as possible. Proper treatment will reduce coughing in two to three weeks and, if the bacilli are sensitive to the drugs used, the majority will be killed within one month. Treatment is needed for a minimum of six months and often longer, with an initial phase in which four to five drugs are used and a continuation phase in which two to three drugs are needed. Because treatment is required over a long period of time and with several drugs, ensuring adherence is often difficult. Another problem in correctional facilities in eastern Europe is that more than half of the people with tuberculosis harbour bacillary strains that are resistant to the commonly used drugs. These people are very difficult to cure and may remain infectious for a long time.

Infection control

The third way of preventing transmission is to reduce the number of infectious particles in the air. The best way is to reduce coughing by providing adequate treatment. But if coughing does take place, simple cough hygiene is very effective. Covering the mouth and nose when coughing or sneezing significantly reduces the number of bacilli in the air (Fig. 8.2).

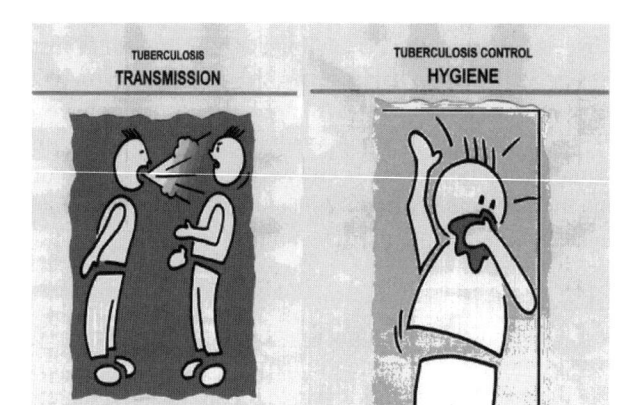

Fig. 8.2. Cough hygiene in Tuberculosis: simple and effective

Source: Royal Netherlands Tuberculosis Foundation (KNCV), 1998.

The concentration of particles in the air can also be reduced in other ways. Ventilation is very effective and can easily be obtained by opening the windows. Ultraviolet irradiation (sunlight) is also effective, but only when sunlight can reach the tuberculosis bacilli. Artificial ultraviolet devices can be used under specific conditions. From an infection control perspective, keeping the windows closed and even blocking the sunlight out by using shutters, as is done in many pre-detention facilities in eastern Europe, is a very bad practice.

Special mechanical filters can be used to filter the air, but in prisons this is not very feasible. To prevent prison staff or visitors from inhaling bacilli, they should wear a special highly effective face-mask when exposed to people with infectious tuberculosis.

Two interventions are available for preventing the development of tuberculosis once a contact has become infected: 1) vaccination with BCG (bacille Calmette-Guérin) vaccine for people at high risk of becoming infected, and 2) preventive treatment for those who are infected but have not yet developed disease.

BCG vaccination has limited efficacy and offers no protection for adults. Preventive treatment can be effective but has a long duration of 6–9 months. Convincing people without symptoms to take drugs for such a long time is difficult. If the bacilli are resistant to the common drugs, preventive treatment will not be effective.

The best prevention in correctional facilities is early diagnosis combined with effective treatment.

Preventing tuberculosis/HIV

All measures undertaken to prevent the transmission of HIV in prisons indirectly also contribute to preventing tuberculosis. Such measures include implementing needle and syringe programmes, distributing bleach, providing opioid substitution therapy and ensuring that condoms are available (for more detail, see chapters 6, 9 and 10). Where the prevalence of HIV is high, people with tuberculosis should be encouraged to undergo testing for HIV and, if positive, offered antiretroviral therapy for HIV/AIDS. Counselling should precede testing (see chapter 7).

People living with HIV who have a latent tuberculosis infection should be given chemotherapy for preventing the development of active tuberculosis. However, in overcrowded prisons in eastern Europe in which the rates of both HIV and tuberculosis are high, this could require using anti-tuberculosis drugs during the whole prison sentence, and the efficacy of the drugs used is questionable if the rate of multidrug-resistant tuberculosis is high.

Outbreak management

In populations with a low prevalence of tuberculosis, the detection of a person with tuberculosis should be followed by screening fellow prisoners, penitentiary staff and visitors with whom the person with tuberculosis has had contact. The usual approach in contact investigations is to give priority to groups with a high risk of exposure (Veen, 1992).

How to manage tuberculosis cases

Isolation

People with tuberculosis should be housed according to infection transmission criteria. People with tuberculosis should be isolated from other prisoners. People with infectious tuberculosis should be kept separate from people with non-infectious tuberculosis. Isolation, however, should not be equated with punishment or solitary confinement.

Treatment

WHO has developed a case classification system that gives priority to allocating resources to individuals most likely to transmit the disease (infectious cases) and to individuals who are severely ill, to prevent death. Priorities for treatment are established according to this classification system. Standardized treatment schemes have been developed, depending on medical criteria.

Treatment adherence
It is important that people with tuberculosis adhere to regular drug intake. Partial and erratic treatment reduces the chance for cure and increases the risk of developing drug resistance. Incomplete treatment also increases the risk of recurrent disease.

Adherence is influenced by the long duration of treatment but also by the possible side effects of the drugs used. In prisons, additional factors may reduce adherence: for example, better conditions in the tuberculosis ward of a prison may induce people with tuberculosis to try to prolong the period of illness, or medicines may be used as an alternative currency. Similarly to the community outside prisons, the health care service should try to increase adherence by directly observing the drug intake and by providing health education and a generally supportive attitude.

Treatment, however, may also be interrupted if prisoners being treated are transferred or released before the treatment is completed. It is therefore important that administrative prison staff members understand the need for continued treatment and work with health care staff to ensure that treatment can be continued upon transfer or release.

How should tuberculosis services in the penitentiary system be organized?

Organization of services
According to Aerts et al. (2006), the justice ministry is responsible for prison health in 68% of the countries participating in the survey[12]; in 14% of countries, the justice ministry is jointly responsible with the health ministry; in 18% of countries, the health ministry is responsible; and in 9% of countries, the interior ministry is responsible. Almost half the countries reported having a system for formal information exchange between the ministries involved in prison health.

In low-prevalence settings, tuberculosis services may be decentralized. A prison hospital may have a special tuberculosis ward. In high-prevalence settings, specific prisons may be assigned for diagnosing and treating tuberculosis cases. A partly decentralized service with case-finding in all prisons and treatment in selected sites or centralized treatment in the first phase and decentralized treatment in the continuation phase may offer the best combination of advantages and disadvantages (WHO, 2000).

Regardless of which department is responsible for controlling tuberculosis in prisons, the prison tuberculosis programme should have the same standards as the civilian tuberculosis programme and use the same guidelines and protocols.

Diagnosis has to be confirmed by bacteriological methods. If prisons do not have

[12] World Medical Association Declaration on Hunger Strikers Adopted by the 43rd World Medical Assembly Malta, November 1991 and revised by the WMA General Assembly, Pilanesberg, South Africa, October 2006

their own laboratories, cooperation with civil laboratories should be sought. Prisons with a many inmates and many people with tuberculosis may have their own laboratory, but external quality assurance is needed.

Treatment may be difficult, especially for drug-resistant cases. If the prisons do not have their own tuberculosis experts, tuberculosis experts from outside the prison system need to consult and supervise.

Treatment, recording and reporting should be monitored in accordance with the national procedures, and tuberculosis cases diagnosed in prison should be included in the national tuberculosis notification registry.

It is recommended that separate departments be created for people who are being investigated, for infectious and non-infectious cases, for those who refuse treatment or default on treatment and for chronic cases. People with chronic tuberculosis often excrete resistant bacilli over a long period of time and pose a threat for other prisoners, health staff and visitors. Strict infection control procedures should be followed (WHO, 2000).

Continuity of care
Prisoners may enter the prison while the health care services outside the prisons know that they have tuberculosis or they may be released while being treated. In both cases, information exchange between prisons and health care services outside prisons is important to ensure continuity of care. This is not only in the interest of the individual person with tuberculosis but is important for the good of society as a whole. Tuberculosis control in prisons contributes to tuberculosis control in the community. The people in charge of tuberculosis control outside prison should be informed well in advance if a prisoner with tuberculosis is to be released, and a tuberculosis nurse should visit this person to establish early contact and mutual trust. Prisoners are often transferred from one facility to another. This may be for administrative reasons, for punishment or on their own request. But regardless of why a prisoner is transferred, the prison staff should ensure that treatment continues. Not only the health care staff but also the administrative staff are responsible for this.

Health promotion and health education
Prison staff and prisoners should receive health education. Overcrowding, lack of ventilation, heavy smoking and lack of general hygiene contribute to transmitting tuberculosis. Promoting a more open discussion about tuberculosis and the associated risk factors (such as HIV infection, injecting drug use, alcoholism or poor nutrition) helps staff and prisoners to understand tuberculosis. They should know about the symptoms of tuberculosis and the possibility of treatment and cure. Both should be encouraged to report people who have tuberculosis symptoms to the health care services for diagnosis and treatment. Providing accurate information to inmates and personnel about tuberculosis and about how it can be controlled will reduce the fear and misinformation about tuberculosis that is often present in prisons.

Monitoring
The prison administration should regularly evaluate the efficacy of the methods

used to identify people with tuberculosis and of the strategies used to contain tuberculosis. This evaluation should examine clinical records, the number of cases identified and the proportion successfully treated but also administrative procedures such as continuing treatment during transfers, staff using masks when dealing with people with infectious tuberculosis and regularly ventilating dormitories.

Occupational health risk

Tuberculosis is an occupational health risk for prison staff dealing with people with tuberculosis. The head of the prison is responsible for undertaking interventions to decrease this risk. These include controlling infection and supervising adherence and providing health education and regular medical examinations. The health care staff should advise on the frequency and methods of regular medical examinations among staff members.

Conclusion

Ultimately, improving prison conditions must be a central component of efforts to control tuberculosis in prisons but also in general society. Most prisoners in western Europe stay in single cells or share a cell with only a few other prisoners and have adequate ventilation and nutrition, and tuberculosis transmission occurs only in shared areas and is relatively rare. In contrast, in eastern Europe many prisoners sleep in overcrowded (and unventilated) dormitories, and nutrition is often poor. Building more prisons helps to reduce overcrowding, but imprisonment rates are often much higher in eastern European countries than in western European countries. Reforming penal codes with the goal of reducing the length of stay in prisons, providing alternatives to imprisonment and reducing pretrial detention times, is a better alternative (Canadian HIV/AIDS Legal Network, 2006; United Nations Office on Drugs and Crime, UNAIDS and WHO, 2006). Large-scale amnesty has also been used in recent years in eastern Europe to decrease the overcrowding and reduce the burden of tuberculosis inside prisons. However, this has increased the burden of disease in the community outside prisons.

References

Aerts A et al. (200). Tuberculosis and tuberculosis control in European prisons. *International Journal of Tuberculosis and Lung Disease*, 10:1215–1223.

Canadian HIV/AIDS Legal Network (2006). *Legislating for health and human rights: model law on drug use and HIV/AIDS*. Toronto, Canadian HIV/AIDS Legal Network (http://www.aidslaw.ca/publications/publicationsdocEN.php?ref=587, accessed 15 September 2006).

Committee of Ministers of the Council of Europe (2006). *Recommendation No. R (2006) 2 of the Committee of Ministers to Member States on the European Prison Rules (adopted 11 January 2006)*. Strasbourg, Council of Europe.

Drobniewski FA et al. (2005). Tuberculosis, HIV seroprevalence and intravenous drug abuse in prisoners. *European Respiratory Journal*, 26(2):298–304.

Martin V et al. (2001). Incidence of tuberculosis and the importance of treatment of latent tuberculosis infection in a Spanish prison population. *International Journal of Tuberculosis and Lung Diseases*, 5(10):926–932.

Niveau G (2006). Prevention of infectious disease transmission in correctional settings: a review. *Public Health*, 120:33–41.

United Nations Office on Drugs and Crime, UNAIDS and WHO (2006). *HIV/AIDS prevention, care, treatment and support in prison settings: a framework for an effective national response.* Vienna, United Nations Office on Drugs and Crime (http://www.who.int/hiv/treatment/en/index.html, accessed 15 September 2006).

Veen J (1992). *Microepidemics of tuberculosis: the stone-in-the-pond principle. Tuberculosis and Lung Diseases,* 73(2):73–76.

WHO (2000). *Tuberculosis control in prisons. A manual for programme managers.* Geneva, World Health Organization. (http://www.who.int/docstore/gtb/publications/prisonsNTP/index.html, accessed 15 September 2006).

Further reading

WHO Regional Office for Europe (2005). *Status paper on prisons, drugs and harm reduction.* Copenhagen, WHO Regional Office for Europe (http://www.euro.who.int/prisons/publications/20050610_1, accessed 15 September 2006).

WHO Regional Office for Europe (2007). *Status paper on prisons and tuberculosis.* Copenhagen, WHO Regional Office for Europe (in press).

9. Drug use and drug services in prisons -

Heino Stöver and Caren Weilandt

Key points
- Estimates suggest that half the prisoners in the European Union have a history of drug use, many with problematic and/or injecting drug use.
- Drug use is one of the main problems facing prison systems, threatening security, dominating the relationships between prisoners and staff and leading to violence, bullying and mobbing for both prisoners and often their spouses and friends in the community.
- The prevalence of infectious diseases (particularly HIV and AIDS, hepatitis and tuberculosis) is often much higher in prisons than outside, often related to injecting drug use.
- Drug dependence services and measures to address infectious diseases in prisons should be equivalent to the services provided outside prisons. This can best be achieved through close cooperation and communication between prison and community services.
- Continuity of treatment for prisoners entering and leaving prison necessitates close cooperation between prisons and external agencies.
- Relapse to drug use and fatal overdoses after release are widespread, and these risks need to be addressed during the time of imprisonment.
- A wide range of drug services should be available to prisoners, based on local and individual need.
- There should be training for prison staff and prisoners on drugs and related health problems.
- Drug services in prisons should be subject to monitoring and evaluation.

Drug use and the consequences for prisoners, prisons and prison health care

Prisons are often overcrowded, stressful, hostile and sometimes violent places in which individuals from poor communities and from ethnic and social minorities are overrepresented, including people who use drugs and migrants. A European study on health problems arising in prison (Tomasevski, 1992) highlighted three main issues: substance abuse, mental health problems and communicable diseases. These three problem areas are closely interrelated.

Although alternatives to imprisonment have been developed and introduced in many countries, more and more people who use drugs enter prison settings. Only some are in prison as a result of conviction for a drug offence. Most are imprisoned for other offences.

Generally, in many countries the number of prisoners has dramatically increased over the last two decades. Several factors have contributed to this, including poverty, migration, violence and the fact that increased incarceration is often politically expedient. Ultimately, however, repressive legislation against drugs in the context of increasing drug consumption in the community has often played an important role.

According to estimates by the United Nations and WHO and information provided by the national focal points of the European Information Centre for Drugs and

Drug Addiction, people who use drugs are over-represented in prisons throughout Europe. In most studies reporting about drug use in prisons, about 50% of inmates report illicit drug use. Between one third or less (Hungary and Bulgaria) and three quarters (Netherlands, Norway and United Kingdom) of the prison population in 20 countries of the European Union plus Bulgaria and Norway for which data are available reported having ever used an illicit drug. Cannabis, cocaine, heroin and amfetamines are the most widespread drugs being used (Klempova, 2006). Considering the high number of prison entrances and releases (turnover rate), a substantial number of people who use drugs go through prison systems annually.

This fact inevitably affects life in European penal institutions. Drugs have become a central theme: a dominating factor in the relationships between prisoners and between prisoners and staff. Many security measures are aimed at controlling drug use and drug trafficking within the prison system. Daily prison routine in many respects is dictated by drug-dependent inmates and drug-related problems: drug-related deaths, drug-induced cases of emergency, increase in the number of people who use drugs, dealer hierarchies, debts, mixed drugs, drugs of poor quality, incalculable purity of drugs and risks of infection (particularly with HIV and hepatitis) resulting from the fact that syringes and drugs are contaminated and shared. Drugs become the central medium and currency in prison subcultures. Many routine activities for inmates focus on the acquisition, smuggling, consumption, sale and financing of drugs.

Prison management is faced with increased public pressure to keep prisons drug-free. Few prison managers talk frankly and in public about drug use in prisons, establish adequate drug services and develop new drug strategies. People who confess that drug use is prevalent in prisons are frequently blamed for failing to maintain security in prisons. The number of prison managers who deny or ignore drug use in prison therefore remains great. Further, many prison physicians believe they can cure the inmates' drug problems by temporarily forcing them to stop using drugs. It therefore becomes obvious why dealing with people who are dependent on drugs in detention is difficult. The goal of rehabilitating the convicts must be pursued, but prison managers in many countries face rising drug consumption among inmates and political and economic circumstances that make solving the drug problem even more difficult. The current situation of judicial authorities is paradoxical. They have to find a solution to a problem that is not supposed to exist: drugs in prisons.

Needle-sharing is prevalent in prisons, but prisoners who use drugs on the outside usually will reduce their levels of use in prison. Many studies from countries around the world report high levels of injecting drug use, including among female prisoners. Studies also show that:
- the extent and pattern of injecting and needle sharing vary significantly among prisons;
- many people who inject before imprisonment reduce or stop injecting when they enter prison, but many resume injecting upon release;
- some people start injecting in prison; and
- those who inject in prison usually inject less frequently than outside but are much more likely to share injecting equipment than are drug injectors in the

community; further, they share injection equipment with a population – fellow prisoners – that often has a high rate of HIV and hepatitis C virus infections (Stöver, 2002).

The high rates of injecting drug use, if coupled with lack of access to prevention measures, can result in frighteningly rapid spread of HIV. There were early indications that HIV could be transmitted extensively in prisons. In Thailand, the first epidemic outbreak of HIV in the country probably began among injecting drug users in the Bangkok prison system in 1988. Six studies in Thailand found that a history of imprisonment was associated significantly with HIV infection. HIV outbreaks in prison have been documented in a number of countries, including in Australia, Lithuania, the Russian Federation and Scotland, United Kingdom.

In addition to illegal drugs, legal drugs (nicotine and tobacco, alcohol and prescribed pharmaceuticals) often contribute to the substance dependence and health problems of inmates. Many prisoners have a long history of regular use of legal drugs. Multiple drug use is widespread among people who use drugs in Europe.

For many prisoners, the first two weeks following release from prison is particularly dangerous, as many prisoners resume (higher levels of) drug use and are at very high risk of drug overdose. Prisoners who have not taken drugs frequently during detention often have difficulty in adapting to the new situation after release. They return to old habits and consume drugs in the same quantity and quality as before prison. The transition from life inside prison to the situation in the community is an extremely sensitive period. The longer a drug user stays in prison, the more difficult adapting to life outside prison will be. Even a prison sentence of only several weeks, during which no drugs are consumed, poses a considerable risk to released drug users: because of a reduced tolerance for opiates, even small quantities can be life-threatening.

In 1988, the WHO Regional Office for Europe (1990) developed recommendations for managing health problems of drug users in prisons. Since then, other efforts to address problems related to drug use in prisons have been undertaken, including efforts to tackle drug users' health problems in juvenile (WHO Regional Office for Europe, 2003a) and adult prisons and the whole criminal justice system (WHO Regional Office for Europe and Pompidou Group of the Council of Europe, 2002). Starting in 1995, the WHO Health in Prisons Project (http://www.euro.who.int/prisons) has addressed issues related to drug use in prisons.

Definition of a drug user
Throughout Europe, prison systems report that drug users are a significant and extremely problematic part of their total prison population, but only a few countries have developed and apply clear definitions of a drug user. Few countries have a comprehensive system to quantify the scale of this problem, even though most countries assume that "drug users" comprise a significant part of criminal justice and prison populations. Several questions arise.
- Who establishes who is a drug user? The doctor on admission, based on certain drug-related symptoms such as abscesses, puncture marks or positive urine testing? Or staff members or the prison administration? Or users themselves

when self-reporting drug use?
- On what basis are people considered to be drug users? Because of the type of criminal offence committed as noted in the prisoner's personal file (violating the drug law and/or other laws in order to finance drug use)?
- Which types of drugs are included? Illegal drugs only or also legal drugs such as alcohol?
- What are the criteria? Lifetime prevalence, drug use prior to incarceration (four weeks, one year?), drug use within prison, occasional drug use, frequency, quantity, setting, problematic drug use, multiple drug use or supplementary use of pharmaceutical products such as benzodiazepines or barbiturates? Which route of administration: injecting, smoking or inhaling?
- Are occasional drug users distinguished from people addicted to drugs?

Nature and prevalence of drug use and related risks in prisons

Drawing a detailed picture of drug use in prisons is difficult in a particular country, and even more so in all European countries. Drug use in prison takes place in extreme secrecy, and drug seizure statistics, the confiscation of needles and syringes and positive urine test rates only indicate some of the full story of drug use behind bars. The patterns of drug use vary considerably between different groups in the prison population. For instance, drug use among women differs significantly from that among men, with different levels and types of misuse and different motivations and behavioural consequences.

The following list summarizes some key information about drug use in European prisons (Stöver, 2002):
- The use of illegal drugs in prisons seems to be a longstanding phenomenon dating back to the late 1970s. Needle-sharing at that time was extremely widespread.
- Substances available outside prison can also be found inside prisons, with the same regional variation in patterns of use. The quality of these drugs is often poor compared with that of drugs in the community.
- The prevalence of drug use varies depending on the institution. Some studies have shown that drug use is more prevalent in large institutions, short-stay prisons, women's prisons and prisons close to a large urban centre. There is less drug use in remand prisons because of the lack of organized trafficking networks.
- In many prisons, the most commonly used drug besides nicotine is cannabis, which is used for relaxation purposes. Some studies have shown that more than 50% of the prisoners use cannabis while in prison. A much smaller percentage reports injecting drugs in prison.
- Several empirical studies indicate that the frequency of use usually declines after imprisonment. This may be due to the reduced supply of drugs or it may reflect the ability of drug-using inmates to reduce or stop drug use while in prison. A minority of prisoners uses drugs daily.
- Imprisonment per se does not seem to motivate individuals to reduce or stop drug use. Reduced drug use appears to be a consequence of the reduced availability of drugs, lack of resources to procure drugs or the fear of detection.
- Some prisoners use drugs in prison to fight boredom and to help them deal with the hardships of prison life or to overcome a crisis situation, such as bad news,

conviction and sentencing or violence. Imprisonment thus sometimes seems to provide reasons for taking drugs or continuing the habit or causes relapse after a period of withdrawal.
- In some countries, alcohol and tobacco are the most commonly used drugs among people admitted to prison or already in prison. In France, one third of new admissions say that they have harmful drinking patterns.
- Many countries report changes in the patterns of drug use (volume and type of drug) when the preferred drugs are scarce. Studies and observations of prison officers indicate that switching to alternative drugs (such as from opiates to cannabis) or to any substitute drugs with psychotropic effects no matter how damaging this would be (illegal drugs and/or medicine) is widespread. Due to a lack of access to the preferred drug or because of controls (such as mandatory drug testing), some prisoners seem to switch from cannabis to heroin, even if on an experimental basis, because cannabis is deposed within fatty tissue and may be detected in urine up to 30 days after consumption.
- Some prisoners use the prison as an opportunity to "take a break", to "recover physically" or to stop using drugs in prison. This time of abstinence is often accompanied by stabilization of general health status (including an increase in weight). Further, many drug users in prisons come from the more disadvantaged groups in society, with a high prevalence of low educational attainment, unemployment, physical or sexual abuse, relationship breakdown or mental disorder. Many of these prisoners never had access to health care and health promotion services before imprisonment. The health care services therefore offer an opportunity to improve their health and personal well-being.
- According to various studies undertaken in Europe, between 16% and 60% of people who injected on the outside continue to inject in prison.
- Needle-sharing and drug-sharing are widespread among prisoners who continue injecting. Although injecting drug users are less likely to inject while in prison, those who do are more likely to share injecting equipment and with a greater number of people. Many were accustomed to easy and anonymous access to sterile injecting equipment outside prisons and start sharing injecting equipment in prison because they lack access to equipment in prison. In the first documented outbreak of HIV within a prison population in 1993, 43% of inmates reported injecting within the prison – and all but one of these individuals had shared injecting equipment within the prison (Taylor & Goldberg, 1996).
- Figures from a European study and some national and prison-based surveys indicate that between 7% and 24% of prisoners who inject say that they started to inject while in prison.
- Some prisoners may also discover new substances while in prison (medicines or tablets) or develop habits of mixing certain drugs they did not mix outside.
- Although smoking heroin ("chasing the dragon") instead of injecting plays an increasing and significant role all over Europe, this route of administration is not widespread in prison because drugs are so expensive in prisons and injecting maximizes the effect of a minimal amount of drugs.
- There is a high risk of acquiring communicable diseases (especially HIV infection and hepatitis) in prison for those who continue to inject drugs and share equipment. Several studies conducted outside penal institutions reveal a strong correlation between previous detention and the spread of infectious diseases. Although injecting drug use in prison seems to be less frequent than in the com-

munity, each episode of injecting is far more dangerous than outside due to the lack of sterile injecting equipment, the high prevalence of sharing and already-widespread infectious diseases. Prisons are high-risk environments for the transmission of HIV and other infections for several reasons, including:
- a disproportionate number of inmates coming from and returning to backgrounds where the prevalence of HIV infection is high;
- authorities not officially acknowledging HIV, thus hindering education efforts;
- activities such as injecting drug use and unsafe sexual practices (consensual or otherwise) continuing to occur in prison, with clean injecting equipment and condoms rarely being provided to prisoners;
- tattooing using non-sterile equipment being prevalent in many prisons; and
- epidemics of other sexually transmitted infections such as syphilis, coupled with their inadequate treatment, leading to a higher risk of transmitting HIV through sexual activity.

- A study carried out in 25 European prisons in 1996–1998 (Rotily & Weilandt, 1999) found an overall prevalence of HIV infection of 5.7%, with substantially higher rates in prisons in Portugal (19.7%) and Spain (12.9%). The proportion of prisoners living with HIV is many times higher than the proportion in the general population (for example, 25 times higher in Germany). Rates of hepatitis B virus and hepatitis C virus infection and tuberculosis in inmate populations are also generally many times higher than in the population as a whole. Where HIV coexists with tuberculosis infection, the annual risk of developing tuberculosis disease is between 5% and 15% versus the estimated 10% lifetime risk for those not infected with HIV.
- Prisoners often regard certain drugs (especially cannabis and benzodiazepines) as serving a useful function or as helping to alleviate the experience of incarceration. Marshall et al. (1999) found that many inmates seem to regard cannabis as essentially harmless. Alongside these attitudes, inmates recognize a need for treatment among those with serious drug problems and were aware of some of the health implications of injecting. They also displayed a possibly exaggerated concern about the problems of drug withdrawal. In the same study, prison officer staff shared many of these attitudes, some commenting on the uses of drugs as palliatives and the relative harmlessness of benzodiazepines and cannabis. Others were concerned about the development of a black market in drugs. In general, staff were acutely aware that the problem of drug misuse in prisons reflected a similar problem in the community.
- Many drug users in prison had no previous contact with drug services before imprisonment despite the severity of their drug problems.
- After release, many injecting drug users continue with their habit. A study (Turnbull et al., 1991) indicates that 63% of those who injected before prison inject again in the first three months after release. Prison therefore cannot be seen as providing a short- or longer-term solution to individuals' problems with drugs.

Prevention, treatment, harm reduction and aftercare
In general, drug services in European prisons can be divided into prevention, counselling, drug treatment services, self-help groups, harm-reduction measures and prerelease and aftercare programmes.

The drug services provided in prison differ widely among various prison systems. Several surveys on the extent and kind of interventions available to drug users in prisons (Zurhold et al. 2005), mainly in the countries of the European Union, show the following.
- Twenty-six countries state that they have a policy related to interventions for drug users in prison.
- Most of the interventions comprise abstinence-based drug treatment (available in 80% of the prisons in the European Union), detoxification, preventing drug use and reducing supply.
- Several countries have established drug-free units and therapeutic communities in separate sections of the prison (Austria, Finland, the Netherlands and Sweden) with the aim of reducing demand. The number of drug-free units is rapidly increasing.
- Methadone maintenance treatment is increasingly available.
- Harm-reduction measures comprising vaccination programmes and the distribution of condoms and disinfectants are available in almost all prisons in two thirds of the European Union countries but are completely absent in the other third of the countries.
- About 19 members of the Council of Europe seem to have a policy supporting pre- and postrelease programmes for drug-using offenders.

Research evidence (Turnbull & McSweeney, 2000) shows that treatment success depends on the duration of the intervention (the longer the intervention, the better the outcome) and its connection with additional services; and the provision of help and support on and after release, with aftercare being increasingly seen as an important component of an integrated treatment programme offered to drug-using prisoners.

Organization and practice of health care, treatment and assistance
Coping with drug use in prison is difficult for several reasons: drug use is illegal. If discovered, it leads to harsh consequences for the time spent in prison such as loss of privileges (such as home leave), segregation, higher control frequencies (such as cell searches) and discrimination by non-drug-using prisoners (fear of transmitting infectious diseases). In the prison subculture, drug users are often perceived to be at the lower ranks of the hierarchy: they are blamed for new supervisory and control procedures that aggravate the custodial conditions.

The prison health service has a dilemma regarding therapeutic resources. Staff of prison health care units and security staff have to deal with the consequences of drug use, but the causes of drug use usually remain beyond their reach. The prison staff and administration often do not have the capacity to adequately respond to the health problems of drug users, especially if they are in prison for short periods of time prisons are not therapeutic institutions. However, the time of imprisonment should not be "lost". The opportunities prisons may provide in terms of health care, social support and involving community health agencies should be used. Prisons can provide an opportunity for helping drug users, many of whom have not had any previous contact with helping or treatment agencies. In many ways, people change the drug use patterns they had before imprisonment, voluntarily or not. Because of a lack of drugs, they might stop their drug consumption altogether, reduce the quantity or change the route of administration because of a lack of sterile syringes.

Most support projects in prisons are designed to induce people dependent on drugs to abstain from using drugs. The objective of making inmates start a drug-free life during detention and after release is probably not realistic, especially because drugs are relatively easily available in detention, and the inmate's past, which was often dominated by drugs, cannot simply be wiped out.

Given that drug use is a reality in prisons, providing adequate services that meet the needs of those affected is imperative. The measures taken must be balanced with the requirements for security and good order. The goals pursued should be pragmatic, not only with respect to the prison system but also with respect to the inmates: harm reduction should be the guiding philosophy behind the measures.

Measures designed to achieve abstention from drug use in prison or at least a reduction of harmful drug-using patterns include:
- counselling on drug-related issues provided by prison staff or specialized personnel with the integration of external drug services;
- housing drug-using prisoners in specialized units with a treatment approach and multidisciplinary staff;
- the organization, methods applied and goals pursued in drug-free units; and
- providing printed and audiovisual material in different languages and involving external counselling agencies in producing this material.

Measures to prevent the transmission of infectious diseases among drug users include:
- communicating face to face: counselling, personal assistance, assistance from and integration of outside AIDS-help agencies and safer-use training for drug users;
- providing leaflets;
- implementing vaccination programmes against hepatitis A and B and tuberculosis;
- making condoms available;
- making bleach or other decontaminants available; and
- making sterile injecting equipment available.

Strategies to reduce risk applied outside prison are often regarded as undermining the measures taken inside prison to reduce the supply of drugs. Supporting the safer use of illegal drugs (such as by providing bleach and sterile injecting equipment) and yet confiscating them is a fundamental dilemma. Studies (Stöver & Lines, 2005), however, show that harm reduction measures can be provided safely and without compromising the measures aimed at reducing drug use in prisons. Harm reduction services complement other measures and provide benefits to the prisoners who are not yet ready or able to stop using drugs completely.

Throughout Europe, treatment orders given at various stages of the criminal justice system differ widely. There are examples of referring drug users from police arrest or remand prison to treatment facilities ("early intervention" in Germany and the

Netherlands in some pilot projects), of putting them under probation in order to ensure that they undergo treatment or of starting a certain form of treatment to avoid punishment before court. Drug users can be ordered to follow a treatment and the sentence is suspended until the end of the (successful) treatment. There are, moreover, several models of community service orders. This chapter, however, focuses solely on treating drug users within the prison setting.

Most countries apply a model of mixed professionals in the care of drug users. External experts are integrated for consultation and therapeutic purposes and to assist the internal professionals in charge of care matters. This type of organizational structure enhances the ties between prisons and the community, to assure continuity of treatment for people when they enter and leave prison. In addition, external professionals from nongovernmental organizations can better guarantee confidentiality and more easily gain the trust of inmates, who often mistrust prison staff, even in care matters.

There seems to be a consensus that prison drug treatment services have to closely cooperate with relevant community services to facilitate dialogue and throughcare (care delivered to the offender from initial reception through to preparation for release establishing a smooth transition to community care after release) for people treated in prison for drug dependence. This can be characterized as a holistic approach. For example, the Moscow Declaration (WHO Regional Office for Europe, 2003b) expresses the need for a close link between public health and the provision of health care to those in prisons.

Prison drug policy should allow for:
- screening, counselling and treatment on a voluntary basis;
- keeping a distance from the drug-using subculture, since drug users who are motivated to undergo a treatment programme have to be able to do so in an environment that allows them to keep their distance from the drug scene in prison, a protected environment, which is difficult to reach for many prisons due to overcrowding;
- throughcare and aftercare, which are essential elements of efforts to reduce relapse and re-offence;
- providing the diversity of measures that are offered outside prisons: social services, drug-care units, drug counselling and treatment services (including harm reduction); and
- discouraging drug import and traffic within the prison system.

Best practice
The counselling, assessment, referral, advice and throughcare services (CARATS) model in England and Wales (United Kingdom) comprehensively links different services that fall apart in some other European countries: prisons, community services and probation. CARATS must be available in every penal establishment via local, cluster or area contacts with community agencies working in conjunction with prison and probation staff. This is a pivotal development for the new strategy because CARATS provides the foundation of the drug treatment service framework, linking:
- the courts and establishments

- different departments within an individual establishment
- different establishments upon transfer of a prisoner
- between the Prison Service and agencies within the community.

CARATS provides a range of easily accessible interventions, including:
- initial assessment upon first reception;
- health liaison with the community on prisoners' reception to prison;
- specialist input into pre-sentencing reports, bail applications and assessments for home detention curfews;
- postdetoxification assessment and support;
- specialist input into sentence planning;
- counselling aimed at addressing drug problems (on an individual and group basis);
- support and advice on a range of drug, welfare, social and legal issues;
- assessment for in-prison rehabilitation programmes;
- assessment for post-prison rehabilitation programmes and drug services;
- prerelease training;
- health liaison with the community upon prisoners' release; and
- liaison with and referral to community agencies to enable effective resettlement.

Beside the development of CARATS, two additional steps of new or intensified drug services have been set up.
1. New rehabilitation programmes have been launched, which include relapse prevention, cognitive-behavioural and abstinence-based 12-step programmes. These moderate-intensity programmes are most appropriate targeted at prisoners who have a documented history of drug dependence and drug-related offending (United Kingdom Parliament, 1999). They have the aim of enabling the participants to reduce or stop using drugs and to address their offending behaviour.
2. Therapeutic communities are intensive treatment programmes for prisoners with histories of severe drug dependence and related offending.

Assessment of drug problems and related infectious diseases
In almost all prisons, the prison doctor sees every inmate within 24 hours of admission for a medical check. Nearly all prisons have a health unit including doctors, nurses and psychologists. Smaller prisons often rely on private contract doctors. The size of the team varies according to the prisons and their capacities. Cases with special health needs are referred to the prison hospital.

Nearly every European prison prepares treatment plans tailored to the specific needs of every prisoner for the duration of the prison sentence, including (formerly) drug-using prisoners. This plan should also cover the measures to be taken after release. Treatment plans include steps towards social rehabilitation and health promotion to strengthen personal competencies and skills. If necessary, treatment measures are included and staff or special treatment boards will review progress. Although throughcare planning is perceived as inevitable to deliver adequate services to drug users, this is harder to achieve but nevertheless necessary for those with a short-term sentence.

Preventing drug use
Developments in several countries have shown that the justice system can play an important role in educating groups or individuals who are potentially at risk of becoming infected with HIV or other bloodborne or sexually transmitted infections. Individuals arrested, detained or incarcerated in police stations, pretrial detention centres or penal institutions can be informed, trained and provided with the means to protect themselves. They are often in contact with help facilities for the first time in their life, even though they have been drug users for a fairly long period of time.

The authorities in most countries have provided facilities at nearly every level of the criminal justice system to facilitate drug users' access to treatment. Since the late 1980s and early 1990s, authorities have been aware of the problems drug users have and cause in all stages of the criminal justice system. Since then, the number of options for counselling and treatment has increased. At every step of the judicial process, the judicial system should ask whether treatment could be a viable and feasible option either as an alternative to detention or punishment or during the prison sentence. Some of these options could be characterized as coercing drug users into treatment by early intervention or while in prison.

Most prisons regard information about the effects of drugs, harm reduction measures and preventing the transmission of bloodborne viruses as a prerequisite for behavioural change or at least a change in attitudes. Some prisons have consolidated social and health care support for drug-addicted offenders, using the first contact during admission with enforcement authorities as a door to treatment or counselling facilities. The admission situation in prison is often perceived as a suitable setting to discuss future plans and drug-free orientation. In countries applying the principle of therapy instead of punishment, the chances of an early transfer into therapeutic communities in the community can be discussed. This is also the first opportunity to hand out brochures, leaflets or other material designed to avoid health damage and to start information and education campaigns.

In Austria since 1998, each prisoner has been given a care pack at the beginning of imprisonment containing an information folder, condoms and a leaflet indicating specific risks.

Detoxification
Nearly all prisons in European Union countries offer detoxification facilities, although they vary in length and form. Detoxification policies vary between countries and often between regions, especially in countries with a federal structure. Many prisons increasingly treat withdrawal symptoms using medication. Immediately reducing the dosage to zero has been replaced with a more pragmatic approach: people dependent on drugs are treated with medication, which permits in-depth analysis of the psychosocial causes and circumstances of dependence. In several clinics the dosage is gradually reduced, depending on people's needs, abilities and resources to overcome or at least cope with their drug problem. Sometimes the detoxification treatments also include psychosocial support, self-help groups, peer support or even ear acupuncture.

The procedures in detoxification programmes vary considerably. In Ireland, for instance, two forms of detoxification are offered: a 14-day programme or an intensive programme that lasts 13 weeks. This involves a support group and counselling. After this programme, prisoners are either transferred to the training unit (drug-free semi-open institution) or granted temporary release. In other parts of Europe, post-detoxification centres have been established, such as in HMP Holloway in England, United Kingdom. This is a community in which residents and staff work together to create a supportive and confidential environment in which inmates can explore drug- and alcohol-related problems during incarceration. It aims to help inmates to become drug-free and cope with staying drug-free, both in prison and on release. The inmates may stay at the centre for up to three weeks. Topics of group work include:

- drug and alcohol awareness
- harm minimization
- sexual health
- dance movement
- art therapy
- acupuncture
- peer support groups
- CARAT assessment
- sleep and relaxation
- stress management
- social skills
- goal setting
- communication and relationship skills.

Prison Service Order 3550 (HM Prison Service for England and Wales, 2000) elaborates clear guidelines to provide effective evidence-based detoxification management for all inmates who misuse opiates. One of the central components is that each prison will have a detoxification service for opiate users developed in conjunction with local National Health Service consultants using evidence-based guidelines in line with the ones developed outside.

Best practice
The Mandatory Task List of Prison Service Order 3550 (HM Prison Service for England and Wales, 2000) includes:

- assessment of needs, which includes the signs and symptoms of drug misuse, and evidence of opiate withdrawal, and also indications that a mental health assessment may be required;
- corroboration of information from the general practitioner, local substance misuse service or dispensing pharmacist;
- urine testing;
- result of urine test to be placed in the inmate medical record;
- the importance of prisoners understanding the need to provide correct information and the potentially life-threatening risk of concurrent illicit drug use during detoxification;
- detoxification guidelines for one or all of the following: methadone, lofexidine or dihydrocodeine; and
- observation by trained and experienced staff, especially in the first 72 hours

of treatment, recorded on documentation kept with the prescription chart or inmate medical record to permit the recording of regular observations.

If detoxification cannot be undertaken exclusively in health care centres, a protocol for sharing information, having obtained prisoners informed consent, with wing staff must be in place:
- staff training;
- availability and guidelines for use of naloxone in the event of the opiate overdose;
- requirements for transfer to hospital in the event of overdose;
- guidelines for the management of those not manifesting withdrawal symptoms and
- referral to CARATs.

Training programmes, in which the staff of prison health care units participate at regular intervals, should provide the necessary knowledge of the latest standards in withdrawal treatments for opiate dependence or multiple dependence and detoxification treatments for alcohol, benzodiazepine and barbiturate dependence. It is advisable to seek the advice of outside doctors who specialize in medication-based withdrawal treatments.

Counselling and support services for inmates participating in withdrawal treatment in prison cannot be effective without the aid of outside drug service providers. The staff in many health care units of prisons have no clear idea about the course of the treatment and do not document the data properly. This applies to examinations of infectious diseases as well as to examinations of other typical side effects of opiate consumption, such as tuberculosis.

Drug-free units
Drug-free units or wings or contract treatment units aim to allow the prisoner to keep distance from the prison drug scene and market and to provide a space to work on dependence-related problems. The focus in these units is on drug-free living. Prisoners stay in these units voluntarily. They commit themselves (sometimes with a contract) to abstinence from drugs and to not bringing in any drugs and agree to regular medical check-ups often associated with drug testing. Prisoners staying in these units sometimes enjoy a regime with more favours, such as additional leave, education or work outside, excursions and more frequent contact with the family.

Drug-free units (often called drug-free zones, such as in Austria in Justizanstalt Hirtenberg) do not necessarily include a treatment element. They aim to offer a drug-free environment for everyone who wants to keep distance from drug-using inmates.

Drug-free units have developed since the early 1990s and in some countries since the late 1990s. In several countries the number of places in drug-free units is increasing rapidly.

Contract treatment units and drug-free units
The purpose of staying in a contract treatment unit is that the inmate will remain

drug-free or at least become motivated for continued treatment after imprisonment. Attempts will be made to motivate the inmate to strengthen his or her health and personality, to participate in work routines and to maintain and strengthen his or her social network.

Before being placed in the unit, inmates have to declare, by signing a contract, that they are willing to remain drug-free during their stay, to submit to regular urine sampling to check for the absence of drugs and to participate actively and positively in the life of the unit.

The unit offers support in the form of close staff contact and possibly relaxed prison conditions for treatment reasons as long as the inmate refrains from taking drugs during the prison term. The contract treatment units work with group therapy and behavioural consciousness. The treatment principles for the contract treatment units reflect a fundamental concept that the inmates can be supported in their decision to stop drug use by offering close personal contact and talks with abuse experts. Thus, a person is attached to each inmate in a contact person scheme in the units. The contact person is responsible for the inmate's treatment plan and for handling general casework concerning the inmate. Moreover, treatment includes sessions with supervisors: external people with a theoretical and practical background as therapists. The contact person, the supervisor and the inmate hold regular sessions tripartite talks to investigate the inmate's development and consider the course of the future treatment. Another part of the treatment is the group dynamics. This consists of motivating the inmates to support each other in the everyday life in the unit. Group dynamics are developed by creating good physical surroundings and an open environment in the units and by both staff and inmates participating in a series of activities inside and outside the unit. Finally, the units work with the concept of the consequential teaching procedure, which means that an inmate caught using drugs or counteracting the principles of the unit is expelled from the unit.

The treatment plans take into account the treatment needs of the individual. They set out targets for the inmates' stay in the unit, and decisions are made on any further treatment outside.

Abstinence-oriented treatment and therapeutic communities in prison
Abstinence-oriented treatment for prisoners is provided predominantly in special facilities (therapeutic communities). Most of the Council of Europe countries have abstinence-based programmes. Therapeutic communities are intensive treatment programmes for prisoners with histories of severe drug dependence and related offending who have a minimum of 12–15 months of their sentence left to serve.

Therapeutic communities are drug-free environments that implement an intensive treatment approach that requires 24-hour residential care and comprehensive rehabilitation services. Residents are expected to take between 3 and 12 months to complete the programme. In general, therapeutic community treatment models are designed as total-milieu therapy, which promotes the development of pro-social values, attitudes and behaviour through positive peer pressure. Although each therapeutic community differs in terms of services provided, most programmes are based on a combination of behavioural models with traditional group-based, confrontational techniques. As a high-intensity, often multistage programme, therapeutic communities are provided in a separate unit of the prison. Many in-prison therapeutic communities ensure a continuum of care by providing community-based aftercare, which is closely connected to the specific therapeutic community and part of the correctional system.

Hardly any research has been done on the effectiveness of therapeutic communities. Any programmes evaluated have mainly been at the local or prison level and are not representative for the respective country.

Substitution treatment
Substitution has become a widely acknowledged and adopted treatment option for drug users in the last 20 years. An estimated 550 000 people currently participate in these programmes in Europe. Substitution treatment has a long and varied history. In western Europe, the first methadone programmes were introduced from the late 1960s in Denmark, the Netherlands, Sweden and the United Kingdom; the 1970s in Finland, Italy, Luxembourg and Portugal; the 1980s in Austria and Spain; and the 1990s in Belgium, France, Germany, Greece and Ireland. Different types of substitution programmes exist, from low-threshold programmes in some countries to high-threshold ones in others.

Already in 1993, the *Guidelines on HIV infection and AIDS in prisons* (WHO, 1993) stated: "Prisoners on methadone maintenance prior to imprisonment should be able to continue this treatment while in prison. In countries where methadone maintenance is available to opiate-dependent individuals in the community, this treatment should also be available in prisons."

The aims of methadone (or other substitution) treatment in detention are to help:
- to reduce the demand (craving) for opiates in detention;
- to reduce the risks of transmission of infectious diseases (HIV and hepatitis B and C);
- to facilitate contact with health care and enable the treatment of other diseases;
- to reduce recidivism;
- to stabilize drug users physically and socially to increase their motivation for participation in further support programmes; and
- to provide a basis for participation in working, education, and training.

More and more countries provide substitution treatment in prisons (Stöver et al., 2004). Scientific studies (Dolan et al., 2005) have proven that this reduces the frequency of injecting among inmates and significantly reduces the incidence of hepatitis C. In addition, the provision of substitution treatment in prison has also been shown to contribute to a significant reduction in serious drug charges and in behaviour related to activities in the drug subculture. Offenders participating in substitution treatment generally tended to have lower and slower readmission rates than people not on substitution treatment. Finally, evidence (Stallwitz & Stöver, in press) indicates that continued substitution treatment in prison benefits in transferring prisoners into drug treatment after release.

However, for prison-based methadone programmes to be effective, a sufficiently high dose of methadone (more than 60 mg) must be provided for the entire period of imprisonment.

Both research into the subjective experiences of inmates participating in substitution programmes and research into the organizational aspects of substitution programmes reveals the heterogeneity of prescription practices and policies in prisons. Short courses of methadone detoxification are frequently experienced as insufficient and inadequate, and prisoners have expressed their dissatisfaction with such a procedure. Scientific evidence (Stöver et al., 2004) strongly suggests continuing substitution treatment begun in the community; adapting the dosage due to the strongly supervised intake situation in the prison setting can be considered.

Very striking is also the inconsistency in methadone prescription in prison compared with the community. The disruption of treatment when entering penal institutions can lead to physical and mental problems and to an increase in injecting drug use and sharing of injecting equipment in prison as well as to an increased risk of fatal overdose after release. Singleton et al. (2003) reported that, in the week following release, prisoners are about 40 times more likely to die than the general population. They recommend providing methadone maintenance in prisons for all individuals with long-standing opioid dependence. In order to meet the requirement that people in prison have access to the same treatments offered outside prison, inmates falling into the following groups should be permitted to participate in methadone treatment in detention:

- those who had already started methadone treatment before imprisonment; and
- those who apply for participation in methadone treatment after incarceration, while in prison, and who meet the requirements for this treatment.

For additional information, please see chapter 10.

Counselling and peer support

Peer education and peer support can be defined as the process by which trained people carry out informal and organized educational activities with individuals or small groups in their peer group (people belonging to the same societal group, such as of the same age or prisoners). Peer education has the overall aim of facilitating improvement in health and reduction in the risk of transmitting HIV or other bloodborne diseases, targeting individuals and groups that cannot effectively be reached by existing services.

Based on the data available and extrapolating from the literature on community-based programmes, education programmes in prisons – as in community settings – are more likely to be effective if peers develop and deliver them. As Grinstead et al. (1999) have stated:

When the target audience is culturally, geographically, or linguistically distinct, peer education may be an effective intervention approach. Inmate peer educators are more likely to have specific knowledge about risk behaviour occurring both inside and outside the prison. Peer educators who are living with HIV may also be ideal to increase the perception of personal risk and to reinforce community norms for safer sexual and injection practices. Peer education has the additional advantage of being cost-effective and, consequently, sustainable.

Inmate peer educators are always available to provide services as they live alongside the other inmates who are their educational target.

Peer educators can play a vital role in educating other prisoners, since most of the behaviour that puts prisoners at risk of HIV in prisons involves illegal (injecting drug use) or forbidden (same-sex activity and tattooing) and stigmatized (same-sex activity) practices. Peers may therefore be the only people who can speak candidly to other prisoners about ways to reduce the risk of contracting infections. As well, peer educators' input is not likely to be viewed with the same suspicion as the information provided by the prison hierarchy. Peer educators are more likely to be able to realistically discuss the alternatives to risk behaviour that are available to prisoners and can better judge which educational strategies will work within their prison and the informal power structure among prisoners. Finally, peer-led education has been shown to be beneficial for the peer educators themselves: individuals who participate as peer educators report significant improvements in their self-esteem (Van Meter, 1996).

However, as with other education programmes, preventive education among peers is difficult when prisoners have no means to adopt the changes that would lead to healthier choices. Peer support groups need to be adequately funded and supported by staff and prison authorities, and need to have the trust of their peers, which can be difficult when the prison system appoints prisoners as peer educators because it trusts them, rather than because the prisoners trust them (Wykes, 1997).

Best practice
In addition to peer education by and for inmates, external organizations operating outreach activities (among injecting drug users) can conduct health promotion. Mainline, a health promotion and disease prevention organization in the Netherlands, maintains contact with detained drug users by low-threshold counselling in prison settings. In individual meetings with inmates, health issues, risk behaviour and the risks of drug use are discussed. An important feature is that as an external organization, Mainline is independent of the prison system and enjoys the trust of the prisoners. Evaluation of their activities has shown: a high level of acceptance among inmates, prison staff and administration; the activity enhances ongoing contact after release; their work is perceived as a valuable addition in the social support structure for drug users; and it is cost-effective.

Harm reduction programmes
A *Status paper on prisons, drugs and harm reduction* (WHO Regional Office for Europe, 2005) defined harm reduction measures in prisons: "In public health relating to prisons, harm reduction describes a concept aiming to prevent or reduce negative health effects associated with certain types of behaviour (such as drug injecting) and with imprisonment and overcrowding as well as adverse effects on mental health."

Harm reduction acknowledges that many drug users cannot totally abstain from using drugs in the short term and aims to help them reduce the potential harm from drug use, including by assisting them in stopping or reducing the sharing of injecting equipment in order to prevent HIV transmission that, in many ways, is an even greater harm than drug use. In addition, the definition WHO adopted acknowledges the negative health effects imprisonment can have. These include the impact on mental health, the risk of suicide and self-harm, the need to reduce the risk of drug overdose on release and the harm resulting from inappropriate imprisonment of people requiring facilities unavailable in prison or in overcrowded prisons.

As shown above, many prisoners continue to use drugs in prison, and some people start using drugs in prison. Despite often massive efforts to reduce the supply of drugs, the reality is that drugs can and do enter prisons.

In prisons, as in the community, harm reduction measures have been successfully implemented in the past 15 years throughout Europe as a supplementary strategy to existing drug-free programmes. Harm reduction does not replace the need for other interventions but adds to them and should be seen as a complementary component of wider health promotion strategies.

The following hierarchy of goals should guide drug policy, in prisons as outside:
- securing survival
- securing survival without contracting irreversible damage
- stabilizing the addict's physical and social condition
- supporting people dependent on drugs in their attempt to lead a drug-free life.

The following text describes some of the most important measures.

Providing disinfectants

Providing bleach or other disinfectants to prisoners is an important option to reduce the risk of HIV transmission through the sharing of injection equipment, particularly where sterile injection equipment is not available. Many prison systems have adopted programmes that provide disinfectants to prisoners who inject drugs as well as instructions on how to disinfect injecting equipment before reusing it. Evaluations of such programmes (Correctional Service of Canada, 1999; Dolan et al., 1994, 1999; WHO, 2004) have shown that distributing bleach is feasible in prisons and does not compromise security.

However, studies in the community have raised doubts about the effectiveness of bleach in decontaminating injecting equipment. Today, disinfection as a means of HIV prevention is regarded only as a second-line strategy to syringe exchange programmes (United States Centers for Diseases Control and Prevention, 1993). Cleaning guidelines recommend that injecting equipment be soaked in fresh full-strength bleach (5% sodium hypochlorite) for a minimum of 30 seconds. More time is needed for decontamination if diluted concentrations of bleach are used. Further, a review of the effectiveness of bleach in the prevention of hepatitis C infection (Kapadia et al., 2002) concluded that, "although partial effectiveness cannot be excluded, the published data clearly indicates that bleach disinfection has limited benefit in preventing [hepatitis C virus] transmission among injection drug users".

In prisons, the effectiveness of bleach as a decontaminant may be reduced even further. There are at least three reasons for this (Small et al., 2005; Taylor & Goldberg, 1996).

- The type of injecting equipment available in prisons, often consisting of whatever can be fashioned into something that pierces the skin, may be more difficult to effectively disinfect with bleach than the syringes used outside prison (on which the studies were undertaken).
- Even when bleach is made available in some locations in prison, prisoners may have problems accessing it.
- Cleaning is a time-consuming procedure, and prisoners are unlikely to engage in any activity that increases the risk that prison staff will be alerted to their drug use.

Bleach programmes should therefore be introduced in prisons but only as a temporary measure where there is implacable opposition to needle and syringe programmes or in addition to such programmes (WHO, 2004).

Where bleach programmes are implemented, full-strength household bleach should be made easily and discreetly accessible to prisoners in various locations in the prison, together with information and education about how to clean injecting equipment and information about the limited efficacy of bleach as a disinfectant for inactivating HIV and particularly hepatitis C virus.

Needle and syringe exchange programmes

In the community, needle and syringe exchange programmes are widely available in many countries and have been proven to be the most effective measure available to reduce the spread of HIV through the sharing of contaminated injecting equipment. Nevertheless, in prisons, needle and syringe programmes remain rare. However, such programmes have been successfully introduced in a growing number of prisons in a steadily growing number of countries including Belarus, Germany, Kyrgyzstan, Luxembourg, the Republic of Moldova, Scotland (United Kingdom), Spain and Switzerland.

Evaluations of existing programmes (Lines et al., 2006; Stöver & Nelles, 2004; WHO, 2004) have shown that such programmes:
- do not endanger staff or prisoner safety, and in fact, make prisons safer places to live and work;
- do not increase drug consumption or injecting;
- reduce risk behaviour and disease transmission, including HIV and hepatitis C virus;
- have other positive outcomes for the health of prisoners, including a drastic reduction in overdoses reported in some prisons and increased referral to drug treatment programmes;
- have been effective in a wide range of prisons;
- have successfully employed different methods of needle distribution to meet the needs of staff and prisoners in a range of prisons; and
- have successfully cohabited in prisons with other programmes for preventing and treating drug dependence.

When prison authorities have any evidence that injecting is occurring, they should therefore introduce needle and syringe programmes, regardless of the current prevalence of HIV infection.

As early as 1993, the *Guidelines on HIV infection and AIDS in prisons* (WHO, 1993) recommended that "in countries where clean syringes and needles are made available to injecting drug users in the community, consideration should be given to providing clean injection equipment during detention and on release". UNAIDS and many other national and international bodies have made the same recommendation. *The International guidelines on HIV/AIDS and human rights (Office of the United Nations High Commissioner for Human Rights* and UNAIDS, 2006) also specifically state that prison authorities should provide prisoners with means of preventing HIV transmission, including "clean injection equipment".

Best practice
Two prisons in Spain introduced needle and syringe programmes in 1998–1999 as a pilot study. Following positive results, nine other prisons joined voluntarily. Evaluation showed the following.
- Implementation in a prison setting is feasible and can be adapted to the conditions of a prison.
- Needle and syringe programmes in prison produce changes in the behaviour of prisoners that lead to less risky injection practices.
- Needle and syringe programmes in prisons help to persuade prisoners to take up drug treatment.
- Implementation of needle and syringe programmes does not generally lead to an increase in heroin or cocaine use.

In 2001, prison authorities issued a directive requiring all prisons to implement needle and syringe programmes as part of the prison regime. As of 2005, these programmes were operating in 33 prisons in Spain.

In Kyrgyzstan, one prison started a needle and syringe pilot project in October 2002. The prison decided to provide injecting equipment in a location where prisoners could not be seen by guards; they therefore took place in the medical wards. The pilot also provided secondary exchange using prisoners as peer volunteers. The project coordinators found that both options for providing injecting equipment were needed. In early 2003, an order was issued approving the provision of sterile needles and syringes in all prisons in Kyrgyzstan, and by April 2004 they were available in 11 prisons. In all institutions, needles and syringes are provided using prisoners trained as peer outreach workers who work with the health care unit. In April 2004, approximately 1000 drug users were accessing the needle and syringe programme. Drug users are provided with one syringe and three extra needle tips. This allows prisoners who inject drugs to inject more – up to three times a day without having to reuse a syringe. This also reduces the cost of the programme, since tips cost less than complete needles.

Transferring harm reduction strategies into the prison setting
Despite the evidence that prisons can successfully introduce harm reduction measures, with positive results for prisoners, staff and ultimately for the community, many are still afraid that introducing harm reduction measures would send the "wrong message" and make illicit drugs more socially acceptable. Many prisoners are in prison because of drug offences or because of drug-related offences. Preventing their drug use is an important part of their rehabilitation. Some have

said that acknowledging that drug use is a reality in prisons would be acknowledging that prison staff and prison authorities have failed. Others say that making needles and syringes available to prisoners would mean condoning behaviour that is illegal in prisons. However, since HIV seriously threatens prisons and communities, harm reduction measures must be introduced to protect public health.

Making available to prisoners the means necessary to protect them from HIV and hepatitis C virus transmission does not mean condoning drug use in prisons. Introducing needles and syringes is not incompatible with a goal of reducing drug use in prisons. Making needles and syringes available to drug users has not increased drug use but has reduced the number of injecting drug users contracting HIV and other infections.

Refusing to make needles and syringes available to prisoners, knowing that activities likely to transmit HIV and hepatitis C virus are prevalent in prisons, could be seen as condoning the spread of HIV and hepatitis C virus among prisoners and to the community at large.

As early as in 1993, WHO (1993) recommended a range of effective activities for preventing HIV infection and AIDS in prisons:
- measures to reduce the number of injecting drug users in prisons;
- measures to prevent drug use;
- information about the risks of injecting forms of drug application;
- information about the risks of needle-sharing;
- demonstrating means of disinfection and providing those means and means for hygienic drug use (alcohol swabs etc.); and
- providing sterile syringes.

Involvement of community services
In the past decade, approaches have developed and grown substantially to divert individuals away from prison and into treatment alternatives as well as a range of services within prisons. Specific legislation in several countries has attempted to enhance links between the criminal justice system and health services to reduce the number of drug users entering prison. Despite this development, the number of prisoners with drug dependence has continued to grow. As drug users often serve short sentences, they return into their communities and many return to their old drug-using habits. Support services need to be continued in order to sustain successes that may be achieved while in custody. This indicates that criminal justice agencies need to link better with drug services.

Prerelease units
Prisoners should begin to be prepared for release on the day the sentence starts as part of the sentence planning process. All staff should be involved in preparing prisoners for release. Good release planning is particularly important for drug-using prisoners. The risks of relapse and overdose are extremely high. Measures taken in prison to prepare drug-using prisoners for release include:
- implementing measures to achieve and maintain drug-free status after release;
- granting home leave and conditional release, integrated into treatment processes;

- cooperating with external drug services or doctors in planning a prisoner's release;
- involving self-help groups in the release phase; and
- taking effective measures in prison to prevent prisoners from dying of a drug overdose shortly after release.

The challenge for prison services in facilitating a successful return to the community is not only to treat a drug problem but also to address other issues, including employability, educational deficits and maintaining family ties.

Harm reduction information needs to be provided to reduce the risk of a relapse to heroin or multiple drug use after leaving the prison. Few prisons speak frankly and proactively about relapse. The prison in Antwerp makes available a brochure for those who leave the prison. It specifically focuses on practical information, health and risk problems (such as overdose) at the time of release.

Many prisons undertake efforts to reduce relapse and to provide social reintegration. Protocols are therefore sometimes set up with drug treatment centres from the national and community health networks. In Portugal, for instance, some projects focus on preparing for freedom and that getting a life means getting a job. Moreover, peer groups are developed to support treated drug addicts to prevent relapse.

Aftercare
Several studies (Zurhold et al., 2005) show that effective aftercare for drug-using prisoners is essential to maintain gains made in prison-based treatment. Nevertheless, prisoners often have difficulty in accessing assessments and payment for treatment on release under community care arrangements.

The following conclusions are drawn from a multi-country survey on aftercare programmes for drug-using prisoners in several European countries (Fox, 2000).
- Aftercare for drug-using prisoners significantly decreases recidivism and relapse rates and saves lives.
- Interagency cooperation is essential for effective aftercare. Prisons, probation services, drug treatment agencies and health, employment and social welfare services must join to put the varied needs of drug-using offenders first.
- Drug treatment workers must have access to prisoners during their sentence to encourage participation in treatment and to plan release.
- Short-sentence prisoners are most poorly placed to receive aftercare and most likely to re-offend. These prisoners need to be fast-tracked into release planning and encouraged into treatment.
- Ex-offenders need choice in aftercare. One size does not fit all in drug treatment.
- Aftercare that is built into the last portion of a sentence appears to increase motivation and uptake.
- In aftercare, housing and employment should be partnered with treatment programmes. Unemployed and homeless ex-offenders are most likely to relapse and re-offend.

Working with families and maintaining family ties
The European Health Committee (established in 1954 by the Committee of Ministers of the Council of Europe) stated in 1995:

One of the inevitable consequences of imprisonment is the temporary weakening of social contacts. It is true that family ties are not broken off completely, in the sense that in most cases a visit of at least one hour per week is permitted; nevertheless the prisoners' relationships suffer enormously from the confinement. A large number of wives, husbands and children of detainees feel punished themselves to a similar extent as their convicted spouses and fathers. Besides, and worse still, in many cases the marriage is bound to fail or be ruined.

Social contacts in general also suffer as a consequence of the imprisonment. In some countries such as Denmark and Switzerland, prisoners are given the opportunity to see their partners without supervision. Supervision is fairly relaxed in Sweden. Working with families of prisoners is a central part of rehabilitation and social reintegration in many countries. In some (such as Scotland, United Kingdom), special family contact development officers are employed to help families to keep or initiate contact with prisoners' relatives, to help to work on relatives' drug problems, to inform families about drug problems in prison and outside and to enhance family visits.

Throughcare
The drug strategy of HM Prison Service for England and Wales (United Kingdom Parliament, 1999) defines throughcare as follows: "By throughcare we mean the quality of care delivered to the offender from initial reception through to preparation for release establishing a smooth transition to community care after release". The aims are as follows:
- to understand the pressures and fears affecting people's judgement on entry to prison;
- to ease the transition process between the community and prison for drug users;
- to provide continuity, as far as possible, for those receiving treatment and support in the community on arrival in prison, on transferring between prisons and on returning to the community;
- to recognize the opportunity that imprisonment offers to drug users to begin to deal with their drug misuse problem, particularly for those with no experience of community helping agencies;
- to ensure that drug users have the opportunity of leaving prison in a better physical state, with a less chaotic lifestyle, than when they entered; and
- to minimize the dangers of reduced tolerance levels on release from prison.

The Scottish Prison Service has general considerations required for throughcare:
- good working relationships and clear lines of communication between prisons and external service agencies;
- drug workers using a partnership approach in prison with their clients;
- encouraging contacts between external agency and inmate; and
- maintaining continuity of care where possible, particularly for short-term prisoners.

Throughcare must involve multi-agency cooperation, which means intensive integration of external agencies that, at the time of release, will continue these efforts. The point of release is vital: how will the treatment work started in prison be continued on the outside, and have the treatment in prison and that available outside been coordinated? The phase of preparation for release should involve community-based professional drug workers. After release, probation officers are involved in further treatment.

Therapeutic communities for sentenced offenders outside prison
Several countries have legal provisions for suspending the sentence of drug users. In Sweden, Section 34 of the Prison Treatment Act states that a prisoner may be permitted – while still serving the prison sentence – to be placed in a treatment facility outside prison. This is not by definition a suspended sentence – it is an alternative to staying in prison until release. Another possibility is that the court sentences a person to probation with contract treatment. This is possible when there is a clear connection between drug abuse and crime. The person has to accept and give consent to treatment instead of prison. If the person interrupts or neglects the treatment, the contract treatment will be interrupted and converted into a prison sentence.

In Germany, Section 35 of the Opium Law allows prisoners to undergo treatment instead of punishment when the sentence is no more than two years. In Greece, after a period of 7–10 months in custody, a drug user may apply to the public prosecutor to continue treatment outside prison, using a law specifically designed to allow drug users to receive therapeutic treatment rather than to stay in prison.

Counselling and the involvement of community health structures
Counselling is a direct, personalized and client-centred intervention designed to help initiate behaviour change – keeping off drugs, avoiding infection or, if already infected, preventing transmission to other inmates or partners – and to obtain referral to additional health care, disease prevention, psychosocial and other needed services in order to remain healthy.

Health care employees require different information than guards or surveillance staff; inmates have their own specific background, subculture and language. Disease prevention material from the outside cannot simply be transferred to the prison setting the relevant target groups require prison-adapted versions. This requires input from different groups based on interviews and focus-group discussions. Initial drafts and design need to be tested and approved. Both prison staff and prisoners greatly influence any prison environment. Both groups should therefore participate actively in developing and applying effective preventive measures and in disseminating relevant information.

Involvement and support from municipal health structures should have priority; nongovernmental HIV and AIDS organizations have especially valuable expertise and networks that can contribute to enhancing the quality of material development and sustaining this as an ongoing activity.

Many Länder in Germany include external drug service providers in taking care of inmate drug users. Some prisons even have their own advisory bureau on drug issues, and the social workers in some prisons take care of these problems. In contrast to internal workers, prisoners more widely accept and trust external workers because the outsiders have a duty to maintain confidentiality and have the right to refuse to give evidence. Moreover, the external workers are more experienced and know about the content of and requirements for the various support services offered. Counsellors on drug issues in prison should primarily provide information about the various support services and programmes available inside and outside prisons. In a second step, their efforts should focus on motivating prisoners to overcome their drug use.

A major advantage of external drug counselling is that it links life inside and outside the prison and thus is very helpful for continuing treatment that was started in prison.

Vocational training
Both doctors and prison staff confront multiple drug use in their everyday routine work. Use of benzodiazepines and opioids is widespread, and withdrawal and craving are relatively frequent. Nevertheless, physicians and prison personnel know too little about issues and problems related to drug use. It is vital, therefore, that staff receive adequate training to tackle the problems connected with drug use in prisons and to move towards a more treatment-focused approach. Prison staff need training and regular updating on all aspects concerning HIV, hepatitis and drug abuse, especialy on medical, psychological and social aspects, in order to feel secure themselves and be able in addition to give prisoners appropriate guidance and support.

References
Correctional Service of Canada (1999). *Evaluation of HIV/AIDS harm reduction measures in the Correctional Service of Canada.* Ottawa, Correctional Service of Canada.
Dolan K et al. (1994). *Bleach availability and risk behaviours in New South Wales.* Sydney, National Drug and Alcohol Research Centre (Technical Report No. 22).
Dolan K, Wodak A, Hall W (1999). HIV risk behaviour and prevention in prison: a bleach program for inmates in NSW. *Drug and Alcohol Review,* 18:139–143.
Dolan KA et al. (2005). Four-year follow-up of imprisoned male heroin users and methadone treatment: mortality, re-incarceration and hepatitis C infection. *Addiction,* 100(6):820–828.
Fox A (2000). Prisoners' *aftercare in Europe: a four-country study.* London, ENDHASP.
Grinstead OA et al. (1999). Reducing post-release HIV risk among male prison inmates: a peer-led intervention. *Criminal Justice and Behaviour,* 26:453–465.
HM Prison Service for England and Wales (2000). *Prison Service Order 3550 – Clinical Services for Substance Misusers.* London, HM Prison Service for England and Wales (http://www.hmprisonservice.gov.uk/resourcecentre/psispsos/listpsos, accessed 15 September 2006).
Kapadia F et al. (2002). Does bleach disinfection of syringes protect against hepatitis C infection among young adult injection drug users? *Epidemiology,* 13(6):738–741.
Klempova D (2006). Trends and patterns of drug use in the EU and drug users in EU prisons. *9th ENDIPP Conference, Ljubljana, Slovenia, 5–7 October 2006.*

Lines R et al. (2006). *Prison needle exchange: a review of international evidence and experience.* 2nd ed. Montreal, Canadian HIV/AIDS Legal Network.

Marshall T, Simpson S, Stevens A (1999). *Alcohol and drug misuse.* Birmingham, Department of Public Health and Epidemiology, University of Birmingham.

Office of the United Nations High Commissioner for Human Rights and UNAIDS (2006). *International guidelines on HIV/AIDS and human rights.* Consolidated version. Geneva, Office of the United Nations High Commissioner for Human Rights.

Rotily M, Weilandt C (1999). *European Network on HIV/AIDS and Hepatitis Prevention in Prisons – 3rd Annual Report.* Marseille and Bonn, Observatoire Regional de la Santé Provence, Alpes, Côte d'Azur and Wissenschaftliches Institut für die Ärzte Deutschlands.

Singleton N et al. (2003). *Drug-related mortality among newly released offenders.* London, Home Office (Findings 187).

Small W et al. (2005). Incarceration, addiction and harm reduction: inmates' experience injecting drugs in prison. *Substance Use & Misuse*, 40:831–843.

Stallwitz A, Stöver H (in press). The impact of substitution treatment in prison – a literature review. *International Journal of Drug Policy.*

Stöver H (2002). *Drug and HIV/AIDS services in European prisons.* Oldenburg, BIS-Verlag.

Stöver H, Lines R (2005). Silence still = death: 25 years of HIV/AIDS in prisons. In: Matic S, Lazarus JV, Donoghoe MC, eds. HIV/AIDS *in Europe: moving from death sentence to chronic disease management.* Copenhagen, WHO Regional Office for Europe:67–86 (http://www.euro.who.int/InformationSources/Publications/Catalogue/20051123_2, accessed 20 December 2006).

Stöver H, Nelles J (2004). Ten years of experience with needle and syringe exchange programmes in European prisons. *International Journal of Drug Policy*, 2003/4, 14:437–444.

Stöver H, Hennebel LC, Casselmann J (2004). *Substitution treatment in European prisons. A study of policies and practices of substitution in prisons in 18 European countries.* London, European Network of Drug Services in Prison.

Taylor A, Goldberg D (1996). Outbreak of HIV in a Scottish prison: why did it happen? *Canadian HIV/AIDS Policy & Law Newsletter*, 2(3):13–14.

Tomasevski K (1992). *Prison health: international standards and national practices in Europe.* Helsinki, Helsinki Institute for Crime Prevention and Control.

Turnbull PJ, Dolan KA, Stimson GV (1991). *Prisons, HIV and AIDS: risks and experiences in custodial care.* Horsham, AVERT.

Turnbull PJ, McSweeney T (2000). Drug treatment in prison and aftercare: a literature review and results of a survey of European countries. In: Council of Europe, ed. *Drug-misusing offenders in prison and after release.* Strasbourg, Council of Europe Publishing:41–60.

United Kingdom Parliament (1999). *Memorandum by HM Prison Service.* London, United Kingdom Parliament (http://www.publications.parliament.uk/pa/cm199899/cmselect/cmhaff/363/363ap02.htm, accessed 15 September 2006).

United Nations Office on Drugs and Crime, UNAIDS, WHO (2006). *HIV/AIDS prevention, care, treatment and support in prison settings: a framework for an effective national response.* Vienna, United Nations Office on Drugs and Crime (http://www.who.int/hiv/treatment/en/index.html, accessed 15 September 2006).

United States Centers for Disease Control and Prevention (1993). *HIV/AIDS Prevention Bulletin*, 19 April.

Van Meter J (1996). *Adolescents in youth empowerment positions: special projects of national significance.* Washington, DC, United States Department of Health and Human Services.

WHO (1993). *Guidelines on HIV infection and AIDS in prisons.* Geneva, World Health Organization (http://whqlibdoc.who.int/hq/1993/WHO_GPA_DIR_93.3.pdf, accessed 15 September 2006).

WHO (2004). *Effectiveness of sterile needle and syringe programming in reducing HIV/AIDS among injecting drug users.* Geneva, World Health Organization (http://www.who.int/hiv/pub/idu/pubidu/en, accessed 15 September 2006).

WHO Regional Office for Europe (1990). *Drug abusers in prisons: managing their health problems. Report on a WHO meeting, The Hague, 16–18 May 1988.* Copenhagen, WHO Regional Office for Europe (WHO Regional Publications, European Series, No. 27).

WHO Regional Office for Europe (2003a). *Promoting the health of young people in custody.* Copenhagen, WHO Regional Office for Europe (http://www.euro.who.int/prisons/publications/20050610_1, accessed 15 September 2006).

WHO Regional Office for Europe (2003b). *Declaration on Prison Health as a Part of Public Health.* Copenhagen, WHO Regional Office for Europe (http://www.euro.who.int/Document/HIPP/moscow_declaration_eng04.pdf, accessed 15 September 2006).

WHO Regional Office for Europe, Pompidou Group of the Council of Europe (2002). *Prisons, drugs and society.* Copenhagen, WHO Regional Office for Europe (http://www.euro.who.int/prisons/publications/20050610_1, accessed 15 September 2006).

Wykes R (1997). *The failure of peer support groups in women's prison in Western Australia.* Amsterdam, Drugtext Foundation (http://www.drugtext.org/library/articles/wykes.htm, accessed 15 September 2006).

Zurhold H, Haasen C, Stöver H (2005). *Female drug users in European prisons.* Oldenburg, BIS-Verlag.

Further reading

WHO Regional Office for Europe (2005). *Status paper on prisons, drugs and harm reduction.* Copenhagen, WHO Regional Office for Europe (http://www.euro.who.int/prisons/publications/20050610_1, accessed 15 September 2006).

International Journal of Prisoner Health, Routledge/Taylor & Francis Group.

10. Substitution treatment in prisons - *Andrej Kastelic*

Key points
- All forms of drug dependence treatment influence the risk of HIV transmission, but substitution treatment programmes have the greatest potential to reduce injecting drug use and the resulting risk of spread of infection.
- The most common form of substitution treatment is methadone maintenance treatment. Methadone has been used to treat heroin and other opiate dependence for decades. The more recently developed buprenorphine is also quite common in some countries. Both have been proven to greatly reduce the risk of HIV infection by reducing drug injection and improving the health and quality of life of opiate-dependent people.
- In particular, methadone maintenance treatment has been shown to reduce opioid use, injecting and needle-sharing.
- Similar to in the community, making substitution treatment available to prisoners has the potential of reducing injecting and syringe-sharing in prisons. In addition, prisoners participating in methadone maintenance treatment have lower readmission rates than those not participating.
- Providing methadone maintenance treatment is therefore an effective strategy for preventing HIV transmission that should be implemented as soon as possible in communities (including prisons) at high risk of HIV infection.
- Methadone maintenance treatment has expanded substantially in the European Union in the past 5–10 years.
- Continuity of care is required to maintain the benefits of methadone maintenance treatment.
- Research has shown that methadone maintenance treatment is more effective than detoxification programmes in promoting retention in drug treatment and abstinence from illicit drug use.
- Before methadone maintenance treatment is started, participants must be provided with relevant information, especially on the risk of overdose and the potential risks of multiple drug use and interaction with other medications.
- Before starting treatment, the drug user should be informed about the primary physician's obligations to the state, to the prison and to the prisoner.

Introduction
There are an estimated 13.2 million injecting drug users worldwide, and at least 10% of all cases of HIV infection worldwide result from unsafe injecting behaviour – in countries in eastern Europe and central Asia, up to 90%.

As discussed in chapter 9, many drug users spend years of their lives going in and out of prison. Generally, prisoners are often from the poorest sectors of society and consequently already have worse health than other social groups. Being in prison commonly exacerbates existing health problems, especially with vulnerable groups such as drug users.

Prisons are extremely high-risk environments for HIV transmission because of overcrowding, poor nutrition, limited access to prevention measures, continued illicit drug use and unprotected sex.
- Injecting drug users are vulnerable to infection with HIV and other bloodborne

viruses as a result of sharing or reusing injecting equipment and drug solution, sexual contact with other injecting drug users and high-risk sexual activity. Although most injecting drug users are men, female drug users may be more likely to use their partner's injecting equipment and often have difficulty in negotiating low-risk sexual practices and condom use. Injecting drug users are relatively more likely to be involved in the sex industry.
- Injecting drug use is now the dominant mode of transmission of hepatitis C virus. Infection with hepatitis C virus results in chronic infection in at least 50–85% of cases. About 7–15% of chronically infected people progress to liver cirrhosis within 20 years, and of these, a proportion will subsequently develop liver cancer.
- The costs of law enforcement, court time and imprisonment together contribute substantially to the social costs associated with opioid dependence.
- On release, prisoners with opioid dependence are at risk of relapse and overdose.

Between 70% and 98% of the people who have been imprisoned for drug-related crimes and not treated during the course of their incarceration relapse within the year following release.

To reduce drug use and its harm in prisons, prison systems should encourage drug users not to use drugs at all; and if they continue to use, not to inject; and if they inject, not to share injection equipment.

Providing both drug dependence treatment and harm reduction programmes in prison is therefore essential.

A consensus is growing that drug dependence treatment can be effective in prison if it responds to the needs of prisoners and is of sufficient length and quality and if aftercare is provided upon release (for more details, see chapter 9).

There are many types of drug dependence treatment, but they basically fall into two categories: substitution treatment and abstinence-based programmes.

All forms of drug dependence treatment influence the risk of HIV transmission, but substitution treatment programmes have the greatest potential to reduce injecting drug use and the resulting risk of spread of infection.

What is substitution treatment?
Substitution therapy (agonist pharmacotherapy, agonist replacement therapy or agonist-assisted therapy) is defined as the administration under medical supervision of a prescribed psychoactive substance, pharmaceutically related to the one producing dependence, to people with substance dependence, for achieving defined treatment aims.

Opioid substitution treatment is a form of health care for heroin and other opiate-dependent people using prescribed opioid agonists, which have similar or identical properties to heroin and morphine on the brain and which alleviate withdrawal symptoms and block the craving for illicit opiates. Examples of opiate agonists are methadone, levo-alpha-acetylmethadol, sustained-release morphine, codeine, buprenorphine (a partial agonist-antagonist) and, in some countries, diamorphine.

Antagonists, which reverse the effects of other opiates, are also used in treating opiate dependence. They occupy the same receptor sites in the brain as opiates and therefore block the effects of other opiates. However, they do not stop craving. If someone takes an antagonist and takes an opiate afterwards, the effects of the opiate are blocked because they cannot act on the brain. If the antagonist is taken after the opiate, the person will immediately go into opiate withdrawal (so antagonists are contraindicated for people who have not been detoxified from opiates). Naltrexone is the opioid antagonist most commonly used in treating opiate dependence. Naloxone is only used for the emergency reversal of opiate overdose situations. Buprenorphine is a partial agonist-antagonist and is being used increasingly to treat opiate dependence. Suboxone is a combination of naloxone with buprenorphine (4:1 ratio) to prevent the abuse of the medication.

Table 10.1. Differences between agonists and antagonists

Agonists (methadone, levo-alpha-acetylmethadol, morphine and heroin)	Antagonists (naltrexone and naloxone)
Substitution treatment	Blocking or aversion treatment
Act similarly to opiates	Block the action of opiates
Stimulate opiate reception	Block opiate reception
Alleviate or stop craving for opiates	Do not produce a rush
Do not produce a rush (except for morphine and heroin)	Do not produce physical dependence
Can produce or maintain physical dependence	

Substitution treatment can be valuable because it provides an opportunity for dependent drug users to reduce their exposure to high-risk behaviour and to stabilize in health and social terms before addressing the physical adaptation dimension of dependence. Substitution treatment is generally considered for people who have difficulty in stopping their drug use and complete withdrawal. It is desirable for substitution drugs to have a longer duration of action, or half-life, than the drug they are replacing to delay the emergence of withdrawal and reduce the frequency of administration. This allows the person to focus on normal life activities without the need to obtain and administer drugs. Further, substituting prescribed medication for an illicit drug helps in breaking the connections with criminal activity while supporting the process of changing lifestyle.

The main goals of substitution treatment
Although the ultimate goal of treatment may be to get people to stop using drugs, the main aims of substitution treatment are based on the concepts of public health and harm reduction. The aims of substitution treatment are:
- to assist people in remaining healthy until, with the appropriate care and support, they can achieve a drug-free life or, if they cannot or want to quit the programme, be in treatment for years or even for their lifetime;
- to reduce the use of illicit or non-prescribed drugs;
- to deal with problems related to drug misuse;
- to reduce the dangers associated with drug misuse, particularly the risk of transmitting HIV, hepatitis B and C virus and other bloodborne infections from

injecting and sharing injecting paraphernalia;
- to reduce the duration of episodes of drug misuse;
- to reduce the chances of future relapse to drug misuse;
- to reduce the need for criminal activity to finance drug misuse;
- to stabilize the person where appropriate on a substitute medication to alleviate withdrawal symptoms; and
- to improve overall personal, social and family functioning.

Evidence of the benefits of substitution treatment

The most common form of substitution treatment is methadone maintenance treatment. Methadone has been used to treat heroin and other opiate dependence for decades. The more recently developed buprenorphine is also quite commonly used in some countries (for more details about these and other substitution agents, see below). Both have been proven to greatly reduce the risk of HIV infection by reducing drug injection and improving the health and quality of life of opiate-dependent people.

Community substitution treatment programmes have rapidly expanded since the mid-1990s. Today, more than half a million drug users receive substitution treatment worldwide. Substitution treatment has expanded substantially in the European Union in the past 5–10 years. Today, all European Union countries have substitution treatment programmes in some shape or form, although countries vary considerably in the extent and nature of the treatment accessibility and quality. Substitution treatment in its different forms has established itself as a widely accepted harm reduction and treatment measure for opiate-dependent individuals in the community (Council of Europe, 2001).

In a common position paper, WHO, the United Nations Office on Drugs and Crime and UNAIDS (2004) stated the following.

Substitution maintenance therapy is one of the most effective treatment options for opioid dependence. It can decrease the high cost of opioid dependence to individuals, their families and society at large by reducing heroin use, associated deaths, HIV risk behaviours and criminal activity. Substitution maintenance therapy is a critical component of community-based approaches in the management of opioid dependence and the prevention of HIV infection among injecting drug users.

The prescription of substitution treatment and administration of opioid agonists to people with opioid dependence – in the framework of recognized medical practice approved by competent authorities – is in accordance with the 1961 Single Convention on Narcotic Drugs and the 1971 Convention on Psychotropic Substances.

Ample data support the effectiveness of substitution treatment programmes in reducing high-risk injecting behaviour and in reducing the risk of contracting HIV. Substitution treatment is the most effective treatment available for heroin-dependent injecting drug users in terms of reducing mortality (the death rate of people with opioid dependence in methadone maintenance treatment being one third to one quarter the rate for those not in treatment), heroin consumption and crime. Drug users have considerable criminal involvement before entering treatment, but the criminal activity is reduced by about half after one year of methadone maintenance treatment. Benefits are greatest during and immediately after treatment, but significant improvement remains for several years after treatment. Reductions are most marked in drug-related criminal behaviour. Many of the concerns raised about substitution treatment have been shown to be unfounded. In particular, substitution treatment has not been shown to be an obstacle to ceasing drug use, and in fact, substitution treatment has been found to be more effective than detoxification programmes in promoting retention in drug treatment programmes and abstinence from illegal drug use. Substitution treatment is a cost-effective method of treatment, comparing favourably in terms of cost-effectiveness with other health care interventions, such as therapy for severe hypertension or for HIV infection and AIDS. According to several conservative estimates, every euro invested in programmes may yield a return of between four and seven euros in reduced drug-related crime, criminal justice costs and theft alone. When savings related to health care are included, total savings can exceed costs by a ratio of 12:1. Injecting drug users who do not enter treatment are up to six times more likely to become infected with HIV than injectors who enter and remain in treatment (National Institute on Drug Abuse, 2000).

Finally, people who are on substitution treatment and who are forced to withdraw from methadone because they are incarcerated often return to narcotic use, often within the prison system and often via injection. It has therefore been widely recommended that prisoners who were on substitution treatment outside prison be allowed to continue it in prison (United Nations Office on Drugs and Crime, UNAIDS and WHO, 2006).

In prisons, as in the community, substitution treatment, if made available to prisoners, has the potential of reducing injecting and syringe-sharing. The WHO (1993) Guidelines on HIV infection and AIDS in prisons therefore recommend: "Prisoners on methadone maintenance prior to imprisonment should be able to continue this treatment while in prison. In countries where methadone maintenance is available to opiate-dependent individuals in the community, this treatment should also be available in prisons." Similarly, the Dublin Declaration on HIV/AIDS in Prisons in Europe and Central Asia (Lines et al., 2004) states:

FRAMEWORK FOR ACTION
Article 1: Prisoners have a right to protect themselves against HIV infection.
Prisoners living with HIV/AIDS have a right to protect themselves from re-infection and/or coinfection with hepatitis C and/or tuberculosis. Therefore, States have a responsibility to provide free access to methadone and other substitution treatments to prisoners in those countries where these treatments are provided in the community. This must include both the ability of people who are already on such a treatment to continue it when incarcerated and the ability to initiate substitution treatment during incarceration. Countries that have not legalized or implemented substitution treatments should do so.

Worldwide, an increasing number of prison systems are offering substitution treatment to prisoners, including prison systems in Australia and Canada, some systems in the United States, most of the systems in the 15 countries that were members of the European Union before 1 May 2004 and systems in other countries, including Indonesia and the Islamic Republic of Iran. In Spain, 18% of all prisoners, or 82% of problem drug users in prison, receive this treatment.

Substitution treatment programmes also exist in prisons in some of the 10 countries joining the European Union on 1 May 2004 (Estonia, Hungary, Malta, Poland and Slovenia), although they often remain small and benefit only a small number of prisoners in need. Finally, an increasing number of systems in the eastern part of the WHO European Region have started substitution treatment programmes (such as the Republic of Moldova) or are planning to do so soon (such as Kyrgyzstan), but substitution treatment remains unavailable in prisons in other countries in the Region. Initially, substitution treatment in prisons was often made available only to inmates living with HIV or with other infectious diseases or pregnant women. Provision generally remains insufficient, below the standards of substitution treatment in the community. In many countries, substitution treatment is still likely to be discontinued when people on treatment enter prison. A treatment gap persists between those requiring substitution treatment and those receiving it.

Some prison systems are still reluctant to make substitution treatment available or to extend availability to the prisoners who were not receiving it before incarceration. Some consider methadone or buprenorphine as just another mood-altering drug, the provision of which delays the necessary personal growth required to move beyond a drug-centred existence. Some also object to substitution treatment on moral grounds, arguing that it merely replaces one drug of dependence with another. Other reasons for resistance to substitution treatment include:
- the fact that prisons are supposed to be drug-free;
- the fear that the substitute drugs may be diverted and sold;
- a lack of understanding of drug dependence as a chronic disease;
- limited space and lack of resources and personnel in many prisons; and
- the cost of substitution treatment and the additional organizational tasks required to implement it.

Some prisoners are also reluctant to benefit from substitution treatment in prisons, either because they lack information about the benefits of substitution treatment or because they want to hide their drug use (one reason being that they fear prejudice and disadvantageous treatment if seen as a drug user), which is impossible if they receive substitution treatment.

If there were reliably effective alternative methods of achieving enduring abstinence, substitution therapy could indeed be seen as inadequate. However, there are no such alternatives (Dolan & Wodak, 1996).

[T]he majority of heroin-dependent patients relapse to heroin use after detoxification; and few are attracted into, and retained in drug-free treatment long enough to achieve abstinence. Any treatment [such as substitution treatment] which retains half of those who enrol in treatment, substantially reduces their illicit opioid use and

involvement in criminal activity and improves their health and well-being is accomplishing more than "merely" substituting one drug of dependence for another.

In recent years, evaluations of prison substitution treatment programmes have provided clear evidence of their benefits. Studies have shown that, if dosage is adequate (at least 60 mg of methadone) and treatment is provided for the duration of imprisonment, such programmes reduce drug-injecting and needle-sharing and the resulting spread of HIV and other bloodborne infections. In addition, they have additional and worthwhile benefits, both for the health of prisoners participating in the programmes and for prison systems and the community.

- Substitution treatment positively affects institutional behaviour by reducing drug-seeking behaviour and thus improving prison safety – prison systems providing substitution treatment benefit, among other things, by reducing withdrawal symptoms on admission (which are often accompanied by self-harm or even suicide attempts), reducing drug trade and increasing the productivity of prisoners on substitution treatment.
- Reincarceration is significantly less likely among the prisoners who receive substitution treatment.
- Substitution treatment in prison significantly facilitates entry and retention in postrelease treatment compared with prisoners enrolled in detoxification programmes.
- Although prison administrations often initially raise concerns about security, violent behaviour and diversion of methadone, these problems do not emerge once the substitution treatment programme is implemented.
- Both prisoners and correctional staff report how substitution treatment positively influences life in prison.
- Substitution treatment offers daily contact between the health care services in prison and the prisoners, a relationship that can serve as baseline for raising further health issues and a linkage with other strategies for preventing HIV transmission.

In Canada, the federal prison system expanded access to methadone maintenance treatment after evaluation demonstrated that methadone maintenance treatment positively affects release outcome and institutional behaviour. Participants in such a treatment programme were less likely to commit crimes and return to prison. This is important because the cost of the institutional substitution treatment programme may be offset by the cost savings of offenders successfully remaining in the community for a longer period of time than equivalent offenders not receiving such treatment.

In addition, substitution treatment may help to reduce the risk of overdose for those nearing release. Many prisoners resume injecting once released from prisons but do so with an increased risk for fatal overdose as a result of reduced tolerance to opiates. Extensive research has noted a large number of deaths during the first weeks after discharge from prison that are attributed to drug overdose. This points to the utility and necessity of prison throughcare of drug treatment to counteract such risk situations and highlights the importance of substitution treatment not only as a strategy for preventing HIV transmission in prisons but also as a strategy to reduce overdose deaths upon release.

Taken together, this evidence – and the importance of providing care and treatment in prisons equivalent to that available outside – provides compelling reasons for prison systems to introduce substitution treatment. Box 10.1 provides an example of instructions for treating drug users in Slovenia (Kastelic et al., 2001).

Box 10.1. General instructions for treating drug users in prisons in Slovenia
- the health services for individuals in prisons or correction houses should be equivalent to those provided outside the correctional system;
- the professional independence of counsellors and therapists is very important;
- close cooperation between the professionals in prisons and in communities must be established;
- addicted individuals must have the option for treatment upon their entry into the prison system (harm-reduction programmes, substitution treatment, detoxification or drug-free treatment); and
- they must have the option to be treated in community programmes.

Effective treatment

In order to be effective, substitution treatment, as any other type of treatment, must be:
- based on the needs of prisoners
- provided for the right period of time and at the right dose required by the particular person
- provided with continuity, upon imprisonment and also following release.

As mentioned above, effective treatment has many benefits for individuals by helping them staying alive; reducing the risk of infection, particularly with HIV and hepatitis; achieving abstinence or a stabilized pattern of use; stabilizing their social life; improving physical health; and reducing criminal activity. It also benefits society by improving public health; reducing emergencies and hospitalization; reducing the spread of HIV and other infectious diseases; reducing social welfare costs; and reducing costs to the criminal justice system.

Substitution treatment programmes vary in duration, dosage and scheme. Although much evidence (Zickler, 1999) indicates that substitution treatment, especially methadone treatment, is more effective when higher dosages are prescribed on a maintenance basis, many programmes focus on short-term detoxification with decreasing dosages.

Applying substitution therapy solely in the form of detoxification restricts its therapeutic potential. Substitution maintenance treatment aims to stabilize health and achieve social rehabilitation. As research indicates, for most opiate-dependent people (WHO, United Nations Office on Drugs and Crime and UNAIDS, 2004),

... the threshold of significant improvement is reached after about three months in treatment, with further gains as treatment is continued. Because people often leave treatment prematurely, and premature departure is associated with high rates of relapse into drug use, programmes should include strategies to engage and keep patients in treatment. Many patients need several years in treatment.

In 1990, the WHO Regional Office for Europe (1990) suggested standard terms for methadone treatment divided into four categories:

- short-term detoxification: decreasing doses over one month or less
- long-term detoxification: decreasing doses over more than one month
- short-term maintenance: stable prescribing over six months or less
- long-term maintenance: stable prescribing over more than six months.

In addition, distinguishing between low-threshold programmes and high-threshold programmes is important. The distinction between these types can be broadly summarized as follows.

Low-threshold programmes:
- are easy to enter;
- are oriented towards harm reduction;
- have as a main goal to relieve withdrawal symptoms and craving and improve people's quality of life; and
- offer a range of treatment options.

High-threshold programmes:
- are more difficult to enter and may have selective intake criteria
- are abstinence-oriented (which could include abstinence from methadone)
- have no flexible treatment options
- adopt regular (urine) control
- have an inflexible discharge policy (illegal opiate use not being consented)
- include compulsory counselling and psychotherapy.

In general, low-threshold programmes are more successful in serving harm reduction purposes for both the addicted individual and society, by retaining people in treatment, which is associated with better treatment outcomes, and meeting the aims of substitution treatment.

Criteria for treatment and treatment plan

Two internationally accepted diagnostic criteria cover drug dependence: the tenth revision of the International Classification of Diseases (ICD-10) (WHO, 1992) and the fourth edition of the *Diagnostic and statistical manual of mental disorders* (American Psychiatric Association, 1994).

Opioid substitution maintenance therapy should be restricted to people who meet the clinical criteria for opioid dependence. However, excessively restrictive regulations regarding criteria for placement in substitution maintenance therapy and its provision that have no significant effect on quality of provided treatment are counterproductive with regard to access to treatment and preventing HIV transmission. Issues such as the maximum dose or maximum length of treatment should be left to the practitioner's clinical judgement, based on the assessment of the individual.

In principle, everyone who is opioid-dependent and in need of treatment should be able to enter substitution treatment after appropriate assessment and treatment induction. In practice, however, treatment places are often limited. In such situations, it is recommended that the availability of treatment places be taken into account when adopting admission criteria. Age, length of opioid dependence, physical and mental health and personal motivation of the opioid-dependent person should all be considered. Some groups, such as pregnant women or people living with HIV or other illnesses, should be given priority. This, however, should not entail compulsory HIV-antibody testing.

For each person, the treatment plan will depend on the objectives of the treatment, which are established based on the possibilities available, the needs and wishes of the person and the professional opinion of the doctor. Issues to consider when establishing a treatment plan include:
- client goals
- current circumstances
- available resources
- past history of treatment outcome
- evidence regarding safety, efficacy and effectiveness.

Opiate dependence is associated with a range of medical, legal and psychosocial problems. A person is suitable for substitution treatment if the individual and social harms associated with the opioid use are likely to be reduced by entering into treatment. Additional problems should be addressed from the very beginning, either by the programme itself or through referral to an appropriate service.

Risks and limitations
The most significant risk of methadone and other opioid agonists is overdose, which can be fatal. Research evidence indicates that the highest risk of overdose is when methadone substitution treatment is begun. Low doses are therefore recommended at the beginning of treatment. However, once a stable dose is achieved (after about two weeks), the risk of overdose death is substantially reduced compared with the risk before treatment.

There are some other negative aspects to substitution treatment. The most important is the fact that, in most cases, a person has to receive treatment for a long period of time. The long-term aspect negatively affects both public spending and the individual person.

The drug user becomes a long-term client who depends on the medication and often also on the person who prescribes it. In some cases this dependence can lead to a passive attitude.

Further, the dependence on the medication and the stigma surrounding it will cause difficulty when people want to move from one place to another or simply travel and take their medication with them after being released.

There are potentially serious negative effects that need to be brought to people's attention before they start treatment so that they can give informed consent to treatment. However, the benefits of substitution treatment clearly outweigh these potential negative effects, both for the individual and for society

Substitution agents
Table 10.2 describes substitution agents.

Table 10.2. Drugs used for maintenance treatment

Medication	Frequency	Optimal dose recommended	Route of administration	Brand Names	Overdose risk	Withdrawal	Notes
Methadone	Every 24 hours	50–120 mg/day	Oral (syrup, tablets) Injectable	Metasedin®	+++	+++	Optimal dose level dependent on subject: it can be <50 mg or >120 mg according to individual variability.
Buprenorphine	Every 24, 48 or 72 hours	**8–16 mg/day**	**Sublingual**	Subutex®	+(with additional drugs)	+	Start 6–8 hours after the last heroin intake or on appearance of withdrawal symptoms. If the person was previously using methadone, methadone has to be tapered until 30 mg/day and buprenorphine can be administered at 24 hours after last methadone dose or on appearance of withdrawal symptoms.
Sustained-release morphine	Every 24 hours	300–1200 mg/day	Oral (capsules)	Substitol	+++	++(+)	
Diamorphine	2–3 times every 24 hours	400–700 mg/day	Injectable Smokable	None	+++	+++	Only available in clinical trials
Levo-alpha-acetylmethadol	Every 48–72 hours	70–120 mg 3 times per week	Oral	Orlaam®	+++	+++	Not available in the European Union
Levo-methadone	Every 24 hours	40–60 mg/day	Oral (syrup)	Polamidon®	+++	+++	Available only in Germany
Codeine			Oral (syrup, tablets)	DHC® Remedacen®	++	+++	Only in Germany for maintenance treatment

Source: adapted from the European methadone guidelines (Verster & Buning, 2000).

In prison, protocols and practices of substitution treatment are often oriented more to the institution's needs and requirements rather than each person's needs and wishes. For instance, the approximately five minutes required for supervising the intake of buprenorphine (sublingual) is seen as excessively time-consuming. Instead, methadone is prescribed.

Drug users may complain about changes in their substitution drug and see double standards with regard to what happens in the community. The prison needs to communicate to the prisoners when replacing one substitution drug with another.

Methadone
Methadone (methadone hydrochloride) is the predominant substitution drug used in prisons and outside. It is a synthetic opioid agonist that has an effect similar to those observed with morphine on humans. Methadone is well absorbed from the gastrointestinal tract, irrespective of formulation type (syrup versus tablet). It has very good bioavailability of 80–95%. The estimated elimination half-life of metha-

done is 24–36 hours, with considerable variation across individuals (10 to 80 hours). This pharmaceutical profile makes methadone useful as a substitute opioid medication, because it allows oral administration, single daily dosage and achievement of steady-state plasma levels after repeated administration with no opioid withdrawal during a usual one-day dosing interval.

Some people experience side effects. The most common side effects include increased perspiration, constipation and disturbances of sleep, sex drive and concentration as well as a potential for weight gain. Such undesirable side effects generally occur at the beginning of treatment and ameliorate over time. In some people they persist over longer periods of treatment, but mostly remain without medical consequences. In total, these side effects affect less than 20% of methadone clients.

Methadone is a safe medication. Contrary to what is popularly thought, it has no effects on bone, teeth or organs. However, detoxifying from methadone is considered very difficult and protracted.

Methadone is inexpensive; it is easy to deliver and the intake can easily be supervised.

Box 10.2. Methadone: the barest basics – a guide for providers
General comments
To the greatest extent permitted by local laws and regulations, methadone should be provided pursuant to the same professional and ethical standards that apply to all other health services. Providers should encourage the availability of a broad range of treatment approaches and sources of care and assist in referring and transferring drug users upon request.

The vast body of experience with the use of methadone in the treatment of opioid dependence should be utilized to the maximum. It is accessible through the professional literature, web-based resources or direct consultation with colleagues. Methadone maintenance – even when provided over a period of decades – is not associated with adverse effects on any organ of the body.

People's lives can be chaotic at the start of treatment, which warrants a relatively greater degree of supervision and structure. Any constraints, however (such as on take-home medication), should be reviewed on an ongoing basis and relaxed or removed as stability is achieved.

Dosage
General: start low – go slow – but aim high
- First, do no harm: estimates of the degree of dependence and tolerance are unreliable and should never be the basis for starting doses of methadone that could, if the estimation is wrong, cause overdose.
- There is no moral value associated with either "high" or "low" doses
- Methadone should not be given as "reward" or withheld as "punishment".

Specific
- Initial doses should not exceed 30 mg.
- Dosages should be increased and decreased gradually. Both for safety and comfort, smaller changes (such as 5 mg at a time) at wider intervals (such as every five days) should be utilized when people are at relatively lower dosage levels (less than 60 mg per day), whereas larger and more frequent changes (such as 10 mg every three days) will generally be safe at higher levels.
- In general, higher maintenance doses are associated with better therapeutic outcomes than are lower doses; the range optimally effective for most people is 80–120 mg per day.
- When there are subjective complaints of "methadone not holding", consider dividing – as well as increasing – the daily dose; this may be particularly relevant for people who are pregnant and/or receiving antiretroviral therapy.

Ancillary services
- The more that can be offered the better, but such service should not be mandatory.
- One of the major obstacles to the effectiveness of methadone treatment is the widespread stigma associated with the illness, the person being treated and the treatment. Drug users should be supported in dealing with this stigma, and providers should seek every opportunity to educate the public (including, perhaps most importantly, health care colleagues).

Maintaining continuity of care
- To the greatest extent possible, arrangements to continue methadone should be made for people upon entering institutions (such as hospital or jail) or returning from them to the community.
- Unless there is unequivocal documentation that higher doses of methadone were given in the previous setting, the dosage guidelines recommended for new drug users should be applied.

Urine toxicology and serum methadone levels
- The value of these and other laboratory tests must be weighed against their costs and the potential benefits of enhanced treatment services the funds could otherwise support.
- Observing the act of urination is demeaning and usually antithetical to an optimal physician–patient relationship.
- Laboratory test results, regardless of how the specimen was collected, should not be relied on if they are inconsistent with clinical observations.

Therapeutic objectives
- Treatment goals might relate to heroin and other drug use, HIV risk behaviour, relationships, employment, housing, etc. – but they should be determined collaboratively by the clinician and drug user and generally not imposed by the treatment provider.

Informed consent – special considerations in drug dependence treatment
- The drug user must be informed at the start of treatment if the clinician's primary obligation is to the state or some other third party – such as to a court, employer, family member, etc. Even if this is not the case, in many countries drug users will not believe that their confidentiality will be protected, and this view – whether justified or not – may affect the therapeutic relationship.
- The drug users must be advised of the specific causes for involuntary termination and the appeal mechanism(s) available to challenge such terminations.
- Drug users considering voluntary termination of treatment must be informed of the likelihood of subsequent relapse.

Source: Newman (2003).

As mentioned above, findings have consistently demonstrated significant benefits associated with both methadone maintenance and, more recently, buprenorphine maintenance treatment.

Buprenorphine
Buprenorphine is a prescribed medication with weaker opioid agonist activity than methadone. Buprenorphine is not well absorbed if taken orally, and the usual route of administration in treating opioid dependence is therefore sublingual. With increasing doses of buprenorphine, the effect plateaus. Consequently, buprenorphine is less likely than either methadone or heroin to cause an opioid overdose condition, even when taken with other opioids at the same time. The effectiveness of buprenorphine is similar to that of methadone at adequate doses, in terms of reducing illicit opioid use and improving psychosocial functioning, but buprenorphine may be associated with lower rates of retention in treatment. Buprenorphine is currently more expensive than methadone.

Buprenorphine is acceptable to heroin users, has few side effects and is associated with a relatively mild withdrawal syndrome. When used in opioid substitution therapy for pregnant women with opioid dependence, it appears to be associated with a lower incidence of neonatal withdrawal syndrome.

Several recent studies (Eder et al., 2005) also report that slow-release morphine is as efficacious as methadone, and the use of a sublingual buprenorphine/naloxone combination tablet (dosing ratio of buprenorphine:naloxone 2 mg:0.5 mg) in opioid maintenance therapy was well accepted and tolerated.

Sustained-release morphine

Sustained-release morphine is seen as a valuable contribution to substitution treatment in some countries (Australia, Austria, Bulgaria, the Netherlands, Slovenia, Switzerland and the United Kingdom). Some studies have reported that the use of oral sustained-release morphine leads to improved well-being of the people maintained on morphine compared with people receiving methadone due to a better side effect profile. In particular, sustained-release morphine is easy to use (once daily), and the users report better concentration, no major mood disturbances, no weight gain and a better drive.

Naltrexone

If a person abstains from opiate drugs, then therapy with naltrexone can be started in prisons before visits outside prison. Naltrexone is a pure opiate antagonist and, as such, is not considered a substitution medication agonist. However, it has recently received considerable attention when used for ultra rapid detoxification under general anaesthesia. In addition to its use as a rapid detoxification agent, naltrexone has also been used for decades as a longer-term blocking agent in maintenance treatment.

The opioid antagonist naltrexone may be used as part of relapse prevention programmes. A single maintenance dose of naltrexone binds to opioid receptor sites in the brain and blocks the effects of any opioids taken for the next 24 hours. It produces no euphoria, tolerance or dependence. People generally require 10 days of abstinence before induction onto naltrexone.

A Cochrane review on the effectiveness of naltrexone maintenance treatment (Kirchmayer et al., 2002; Minozzi et al., 2006) did not find evidence for its effectiveness in maintenance therapy. However, a trend in favour of treatment with naltrexone was observed for certain target groups (especially people who are highly motivated).

The effectiveness of naltrexone treatment clearly hinges on compliance with treatment and the motivation to take the medication each day.

Some basic information about treatment

Information users require

The absolute condition for an effective start of substitution treatment is to provide the user with relevant information, in particular on the risk of overdose, which should include the following:
- the delay of a peak effect of the substitute drug (methadone 2–4 hours);

- the accumulation of the substitution drug over time resulting in a greater effect (methadone over 3–5 days or more), even on a fixed dose;
- the risks of multiple drug use while in substitution treatment, especially other opiates, cocaine, benzodiazepines and alcohol; and
- the potential interaction with other medication.

In addition, users need information about substitution treatment and drugs in general and about particular rules and expectations. Prisoners often do not understand the goals pursued with the substitution treatment, nor do they have enough information about the specific drug used or the rules they have to follow. Prisoners should be asked to sign an informed consent form once they have clearly understood all relevant information.

Anonymity and confidentiality of treatment
Every prisoner should know before getting any sort of treatment the primary physician's obligation: to the state, to the prison or to the prisoner.

Although securing anonymity and confidentiality within a prison is difficult, attempts have been made to administer substitution drugs in a way that protects prisoners, either by putting all drug users together in one wing or delivering substitution drugs discreetly with other pharmaceuticals.

Other inmates and staff should not be made aware that a prisoner is a drug user or in substitution treatment. The fear is that if somebody knows about the drug dependence, it will lead to consequences for the actual sentence in terms of disadvantages (such as access to work, qualification or jobs), prejudices, loss of privileges or simply the negative attitude of staff and other prisoners. Moreover, the drug users fear pressure from other inmates who wish to participate in the substitution treatment in terms of smuggling substitution drugs.

However, informing properly trained guards and other staff involved in work with the prisoner can be useful. Shutting guards completely out of the psychosocial and health care support also seems to build barriers between the different professionals and sometimes enhances prejudices and misunderstandings about the prisoner and drug use. Hence, basic cooperation, information and training of prison staff, including guards, are needed to ensure that staff members have positive or at least better attitudes towards drug users.

Privileges
Patients on substitution treatment who follow the rules in their therapeutic agreement should be able to enjoy all the same privileges as other prisoners. Decisions regarding flexible release should be made based on the therapist's individual judgement. Flexible releases should be planned and performed gradually.

Take-home dosages can be given as privileges for visits or holidays outside prison that are longer than 24 hours. The prisoner receiving the substitution treatment must be able to continue with such treatment and must have the possibility of being included in other programmes after release. The physician decides about ability to work.

Users' involvement
Ongoing contributions from drug users are valuable in order to improve the quality of health care; most prisoners have had previous, personal experience of prison health care and substitution treatment inside prison and in the community (either detoxification or maintenance).

Acknowledging and integrating prisoner's experiences and expertise in involving drug users in developing, designing and delivering interventions is critical to increasing their appropriateness and reach.

Support groups or educational programmes should be established or incorporated into the overall HIV treatment programme for injecting drug users. Former injecting drug users often have unique success in educating and motivating current injecting drug users to take steps to access effective care.

The link with treatment for HIV infection
Substitution treatment offers opportunities for improving the delivery of antiretroviral therapy to opioid users living with HIV. Substitution treatment enables opioid-dependent drug users to stabilize their lives and avoid or manage many of the complications of injecting drug use. It is therefore seen as an essential component in strategies for retaining active injecting drug users in treatment. It also provides additional entry points for scaling up antiretroviral therapy, improves drug adherence and increases access to care.

Substitution treatment programmes can be of great importance to injecting drug users living with HIV by:
- offering HIV testing for injecting drug users;
- referring them to HIV services;
- liaising with HIV services regarding treatment and care;
- preparing injecting drug users for treatment with antiretroviral therapy;
- dispensing antiretroviral therapy in conjunction with opioid substitution treatment;
- monitoring and managing the side effects of antiretroviral therapy;
- monitoring and managing interaction between methadone or buprenorphine and antiretroviral therapy; and
- supporting individual and family through the lifelong commitment to antiretroviral therapy.

This daily contact with substitution treatment programmes has potentially huge advantages for access and adherence to antiretroviral therapy.

Special considerations for women
Women tend to have a different experience than men with both drug dependence and treatment. Major issues are related to the high levels of both physical and mental co-morbidity of women with opioid dependence, and these need to be taken into account in providing treatment. Women with opioid dependence often face a variety of barriers to treatment, including lack of financial resources, absence of services and referral networks oriented to women and conflicting child-care responsibilities.

Effective substitution treatment of opioid dependence can substantially improve obstetric, parental and neonatal outcomes. Opioid substitution maintenance therapy also has an important role in attracting and retaining pregnant women in treatment and ensuring good contact with obstetric and community-based services, including primary care.

Future perspectives
In order to ensure that prisons provide a level of care equivalent to that provided outside, (1) a major expansion of care for sexually transmitted infections is needed in many countries to meet the needs of prisoners, (2) substantial efforts have to be made to improve the quality of services and (3) better links and continuity of care are needed between prisons and the range of community-based services.

The 2002 Consensus Statement on Prisons, Drugs, and Society (WHO Regional Office for Europe and Pompidou Group of the Council of Europe, 2002) recognizes that:
- drugs and prisons have to be seen in the wider social context
- people move between prisons and the community
- imprisonment should not mean more punishment than the deprivation of liberty
- prisons must be safe, secure and decent places in which people live and work
- people working in prisons must work within the law as it stands.

Given the existing evidence of the growing problems of injecting drug use and HIV/AIDS in prisons and of the effectiveness of substitution treatment, the time to act is clearly now. Failure to implement effective drug treatment, including substitution treatment, and measures to prevent HIV transmission will result in further spread of HIV infection among injecting drug users, the larger prison population, and ultimately, in the community outside prisons.

References
American Psychiatric Association (1994). *Diagnostic and statistical manual of mental disorders.* Washington, DC, American Psychiatric Association.
Council of Europe (2001). *11th general report on the CPT's activities covering the period 1 January to 31 December 2000.* Strasbourg, Council of Europe, 2001 (CPT/Inf (2001) 16).
Dolan KA, Wodak AD, Hall WD (1996). An international review of methadone provision in prisons. *Addiction Research*, 4:85–97.
Eder H et al. (2005). Comparative study of the effectiveness of slow-release morphine and methadone for opioid maintenance therapy. *Addiction*, 100:1101–1109.
Kirchmayer U et al. (2002). A systematic review on the efficacy of naltrexone maintenance treatment in opioid dependence. *Addiction*, 97:1241–1249.
Kastelic A, Perhavc O, Kostnapfel Rihtar T (2001). *General instructions for treating drug users in prisons in Slovenia.* Ljubljana, Ministry of Health of the Republic of Slovenia, Ministry of Justice of the Republic of Slovenia, 2001.
Lines R et al. (2004). *Dublin Declaration on HIV/AIDS in Prisons in Europe and Central Asia.* Dublin, Irish Penal Reform Trust.
Minozzi S et al. (2006). Oral naltrexone maintenance treatment for opioid depend-

ence. *Cochrane Database of Systematic Reviews*, (1):CD001333.
National Institute on Drug Abuse (2000). *Principles of drug addiction treatment: a research based guide*. Bethesda, MD, National Institute on Drug Abuse.
Newman R (2003). Methadone: the barest basics; a guide for providers. *SEEA Addictions*, 4(1–2).
United Nations Office on Drugs and Crime, UNAIDS and WHO (2006). *HIV/AIDS prevention, care, treatment and support in prison settings: a framework for an effective national response*. Vienna, United Nations Office on Drugs and Crime (http://www.who.int/hiv/treatment/en/index.html, accessed 15 September 2006).
Verster A, Buning E (2000). *European methadone guidelines*. Amsterdam, EuroMethwork (http://www.q4q.nl/methwork/startguidelines.htm, accessed 15 September 2006).
WHO (1993). *Guidelines on HIV infection and AIDS in prisons*. Geneva, World Health Organization, 1993 (http://whqlibdoc.who.int/hq/1993/WHO_GPA_DIR_93.3.pdf, accessed 15 September 2006).
WHO, United Nations Office on Drugs and Crime, UNAIDS (2004). *Substitution maintenance therapy in the management of opioid dependence and HIV/AIDS prevention*. Geneva, World Health Organization (http://www.who.int/substance_abuse/publications/psychoactives/en/index.html, accessed 15 September 2006).
WHO Regional Office for Europe (1990). *Drug abusers in prisons: managing their health problems. Report on a WHO meeting, The Hague, 16–18 May 1988*. Copenhagen, WHO Regional Office for Europe (WHO Regional Publications, European Series, No. 27).
WHO Regional Office for Europe, Pompidou Group of the Council of Europe (2002). *Prisons, drugs and society*. Copenhagen, WHO Regional Office for Europe (http://www.euro.who.int/prisons/publications/20050610_1, accessed 15 September 2006).

Further reading
Anonymous (2005). Prison health: a threat or an opportunity? *Lancet*, 366:57.
Council of Europe (2001). *Development and improvement of substitution programmes*. Strasbourg, Council of Europe Publishing.
European Monitoring Centre for Drugs and Drug Addiction (2002). Key role of substitution in drug treatment. *Drugs in Focus*, Issue 1 (January-February) (http://www.emcdda.europa.eu/?nnodeid=439, accessed 15 September 2006).
European Monitoring Centre for Drugs and Drug Addiction (2003). Treating drug users in prison – a critical area for health-promotion and crime-reduction policy. *Drugs in Focus*, Issue 7 (January-February) (http://www.emcdda.europa.eu/?nnodeid=439, accessed 15 September 2006).
Ford C et al. (2003). *Guidance for the use of buprenorphine for the treatment of opioid dependence in primary care*. London, RCGP Drug and Alcohol Misuse Training Programme, RCGP Sex, Drugs and HIV Task Group and SMMGP (http://www.smmgp.org.uk/html/guidance.php, accessed 15 September 2006)).
Kastelic A (2004). Statement on the 7th European Conference on Drug and HIV/AIDS Services in Prison, "Prison, Drugs and Society in the Enlarged Europe". In: Stöver H, Hennebel LC, Casselmann J, eds. *Substitution treatment in European prisons. A study of policies and practices if substitution in prisons in 18 European countries*. London, European Network of Drug Services in Prison.
Kastelic A, Kostnapfel Rihtar T (2003). Drug addiction treatment in the Republic of Slovenia. *SEEA Addictions*, 4(1–2).

Kastelic A, Perhavc O, Kostnapfel Rihtar T (2001). *General instructions for treating drug users in prisons in Slovenia.* Ljubljana, Ministry of Health of the Republic of Slovenia, Ministry of Justice of the Republic of Slovenia, 2001.

Kerr T, Jürgens R (2004). *Methadone maintenance therapy in prisons: reviewing the evidence.* Montreal, Canadian HIV/AIDS Legal Network (http://pubs.cpha.ca/PDF/P31/22907.pdf, accessed 15 September 2006).

Kraigher D et al. (2005). Use of slow-release oral morphine for the treatment of opioid dependence. *European Addiction Research,* 11:145–151.

La Vincente S (in press). *Treatment of injecting drug users with HIV/AIDS: promoting access and optimizing service delivery.* Geneva, World Health Organization.

MacDonald M (2004). *A study of existing drug services and strategies operating in prisons in ten countries from central and eastern Europe.* Warsaw, Central and Eastern European Network of Drug Services in Prison (CEENDSP), Cranstoun Drug Services (http://www.endipp.net/index.php?option=com_remository&Itemid=42&func=selectcat&cat=1, accessed 15 September 2006).

National Institute on Drug Abuse (2000). *Principles of drug addiction treatment: a research based guide.* Bethesda, MD, National Institute on Drug Abuse.

Newman R. (2003). Methadone: the barest basics; a guide for providers. *SEEA Addiction,* 4:1–2.

Stöver H, Casselman J, Hennebel L (2006). Substitution treatment in European prisons: a study of policy and practices in 18 European countries. *International Journal of Prison Health,* 2:3–12.

Uchtenhagen A (2002). Drug abuse treatment in the prison milieu: a review of the evidence. In: Council of Europe, ed. *Prisons, drugs and society.* Strasbourg, Council of Europe:79–98.

United Nations Office on Drugs and Crime (2002). *Contemporary drug abuse treatment: a review of the evidence base.* Vienna, United Nations Office on Drugs and Crime (http://www.unodc.org/unodc/treatment_toolkit.html. accessed 15 September 2006).

United Nations Office on Drugs and Crime (2003). *Investing in drug abuse treatment: a discussion paper for policy makers.* Vienna, United Nations Office on Drugs and Crime. (http://www.unodc.org/unodc/treatment_toolkit.html. accessed 15 September 2006).

Verster A, Buning E (2003). *Information for policymakers on the effectiveness of substitution treatment for opiate dependence.* Amsterdam, EuroMethwork.

Verster A, Buning E. *Key aspects of substitution treatment for opiate dependence.* Amsterdam, EuroMethwork 2003.

Verster A, Keenan E (2005). *HIV/AIDS treatment and care protocols for injecting drug users:* draft. Lisbon, WHO Technical Consultation, in collaboration with EMCDDA, on the Development of HIV/AIDS Treatment and Care Protocols for IDU, 2005.

WHO (2004). *The practices and context of pharmacotherapy of opioid dependence in central and eastern Europe.* Geneva, World Health Organization (http://www.who.int/substance_abuse/publications/treatment/en/index.html, accessed 15 September 2006).

WHO Regional Office for Europe (2005). *Status paper on prisons, drugs and harm reduction.* Copenhagen, WHO Regional Office for Europe (http://www.euro.who.int/prisons/publications/20050610_1, accessed 15 September 2006).

Zickler P (1999). High-dose methadone improves treatment outcomes. *NIDA Notes,* 14(5) (http://www.nida.nih.gov/NIDA_Notes/NNVol14N5/HighDose.html, accessed 21 December 2006).

11. Mental health in prisons -

Eric Blaauw and Hjalmar J.C. van Marle

Key points
- Mental disorders and suicide are highly prevalent in prisons.
- Several factors associated with imprisonment are intrinsically hazardous for the mental health of prisoners.
- Prisoners should receive the same level and quality of basic health services as in the community (equivalence principle).
- It is vital that prisons cooperate with community agencies to secure equality and continuity of treatment.
- About 6–12% of all prisoners need to be transferred to specialized institutions, 30–50% need assistance from health care services and 40–60% would benefit most from mental health promotion. Consequently, different levels of care are required.
- Forensic health care should be available on a continuous basis to prevent the deterioration of the mental health state of the prisoners, and forensic psychiatric care should be available for those prisoners who need it. Specialized psychiatric treatment (forensic psychiatric treatment) may be necessary to decrease the chance of recidivism.
- The presence of health care personnel does not guarantee good mental health. Maintaining good detention circumstances provides a further safeguard against the deterioration of mental health and promotes mental health. For this, adhering to the United Nations Standard Minimum Rules for the Treatment of Prisoners is important.
- The best safeguard is in place when all prison personnel are carefully selected and adequately trained in reducing mental harm and promoting mental health.

Mental health and mental illness in prisons

About nine million people are detained in penal institutions around the world. At least half of these struggle with personality disorders, and one million prisoners or more worldwide suffer from serious mental disorders such as psychosis or depression. Nearly all prisoners experience depressed moods or stress symptoms. Moreover, each year several thousand prisoners take their own lives during imprisonment.

About 4% of male and female prisoners have psychotic illnesses, 10% (men) to 12% (women) have major depression, and 42% (women) to 65% (men) have a personality disorder, including 21% (women) to 47% (men) with antisocial personality disorder (Fazel & Danesh, 2002). Research (Blaauw et al., 1998) has also shown that 89% of all prisoners have depressive symptoms and 74% have stress-related somatic symptoms. Thus, imprisonment is clearly associated with mental health problems among those who are subjected to it.

Many people with mental disorders are arrested and imprisoned, causing mental problems to be imported from the outside world into the prisons. In other cases, people without mental disorders develop mental problems during their imprisonment due to the deprivation they encounter in the prisons.
Certain types of deprivation are inevitable in prisons. For instance, prisoners are deprived of their liberty for a period that may be long or of uncertain length.

Deprivation of liberty inevitably involves deprivation of choices taken for granted in the outside community. They can no longer freely decide where to live, with whom to associate and how to fill their time and must submit to discipline imposed by others. Communication with families and friends is limited and often without privacy.

Other factors that often apply in prisons and that could adversely affect mental health include overcrowding, dirty and depressing environments, poor food, inadequate health care, aggression (which may take many forms, such as physical, verbal, racial or sexual), lack of purposeful activity, the availability of illicit drugs and either enforced solitude or lack of privacy and time for quiet relaxation and reflection.

Further, prisoners may have feelings of guilt or shame about the offences they have committed, the fact that they have been imprisoned and the effects of their behaviour on other people, including their families and friends, coupled with anxiety about how much of their former lives will remain intact after release. Prisoners seeking asylum or awaiting removal to another country face additional anxiety and may feel particularly isolated.

The cumulative effect of all these factors, left unchecked, is to worsen the mental health of prisoners and to increase the likelihood of incidents damaging to the wellbeing of prisoners and staff, as well as to good order and security, such as displays of aggression, bullying, mobbing, suicide attempts and self-harm. In prisons experiencing high levels of such incidents, staff and prisoners suffer the effects of increased tension, with consequent ill effects on their mental health. Thus, prisoners as well as staff benefit from reducing mental harm and promoting mental health in prisons.

Mental health is a positive sense of well-being, from which springs the emotional and spiritual resilience that is important for personal fulfilment and enables people to survive pain, disappointment and sadness (WHO Regional Office for Europe, 1999). It requires an underlying belief in our own and others' dignity and worth. Although contemplating the existence of positive mental health among prisoners may be difficult, prison should provide an opportunity for prisoners to be helped towards a sense of the opportunities available to them for personal development, without harming themselves or others.

Mental harm reduction and mental health promotion
The main principle in penal law is that the prison sentence is the essential sentence: that is, prison sentences should be sufficient punishment for the prisoner and should be sufficient for society. Discipline, order and instruments of restraint (such as handcuffs, chains and straitjackets) as well as other aspects of prison sentences may have real disadvantages in prisoners' experiences, lack of freedom and the atmosphere in which they are kept, but they should never have the character of another punishment.

In forensic ethics regarding prison health care, the aim has to be to implement health care in the prison based on the principle of equivalence. This means that the level and quality of the basic health services should be the same as in the community. In addition, when further specialized medical examinations, interventions and aftercare are needed, these should be applied in a special part of the prison in ways that are equal to how they are applied in the community. In this way the demands of public protection are not breached. If the health condition of the prisoner necessitates it, the detainee has the right to be transferred to a hospital under custody. The necessary treatment cannot be withdrawn, which is why many countries have prison hospitals to which prisoners can be transferred for treatment in which health care can be provided in safe and guarded surroundings.

Having recognized the afore-mentioned problems and based on the principle of equality, the WHO consensus statement (WHO Regional Office for Europe, 1999) says:

In order to achieve positive mental health, countries must have in place positive mental health legislation, close integration of health, penal and social policy and effective aftercare following imprisonment. Prisoners remain members of the community; therefore prisons should work in partnership with prisoners, their families and appropriate community agencies to deliver programmes and treatment that engage those in prison with the community at an early stage of any period in custody. Cooperation with community agencies is vital to secure continuity of treatment (for example, treatment of psychiatric illness and substance abuse) and to facilitate the reintegration of the prisoner into the community.

In addition, the WHO European Health in Prisons Project strongly recommends that all prison authorities, health authorities and prison staff recognize and seize all the opportunities the prison setting presents to eliminate or reduce the mental harm imprisonment may cause and to promote mental health. Governments and authorities responsible for all forms of compulsory detention are invited to consider the relevance of the WHO consensus statement (WHO Regional Office for Europe, 1999) to their local circumstances and to adopt its provisions, implementing them in accordance with national legal requirements. In this respect, the Committee of Ministers of the Council of Europe (1998) stated that respect for the fundamental rights of prisoners entails the provision to prisoners of preventive treatment and health care equivalent to those provided to the community in general. This could mean that mental health services should follow the same principles as endorsed at the Helsinki Declaration in 2005 (WHO 2005).

Levels of care

Not all prisoners with mental disorders need specialist psychiatric treatment. Research (Blaauw et al., 2000) suggests that the need for transfer for further assessment and treatment of prisoners with mental disorders is met when 6–12% of a country's prison population can be transferred. An additional 30–50% of all prisoners do not need transfer or urgent psychiatric attention but do need some assistance from health care services (see below). The remaining 40–60% would benefit most from mental health promotion. The question is, however, what is psychiatric treatment, what is assistance by health care services and what is mental health promotion? In other words: which levels of care exist and what are their characteristics?

All prisons need sufficient support to counterbalance the destabilizing negative influences of prison circumstances. Forensic health care (Ministry of Justice, the Netherlands, 2003) is needed that should be available on a continuous basis in the prison itself, in addition to the basic health care, and with a primary aim of preventing the mental health of the prisoners from deteriorating due to the prison atmosphere. Moreover, forensic health care is often necessary due to the presence of very vulnerable detainees (such as drug-dependent people, psychiatric patients and estranged people) and the unique characteristics of the situation (such as a strict hierarchy of correctional officers). The United Nations[13] has formulated a Standard Minimum Rule for this (Rule 22), which states (Office of the United Nations High Commissioner for Human Rights, 1957):

At every institution there shall be available the services of at least one qualified medical officer who should have some knowledge of psychiatry. The medical services should be organized in close relationship to the general health administration of the community or nation. They shall include a psychiatric service for the diagnosis and, in proper cases, the treatment of states of mental abnormality.

It is justifiable that the difficult prison circumstances require that a psychologist also take part in the fundamental basic care. Next to a prison doctor, nurses and a psychologist, there is also the need for consultation of a psychiatrist, a social worker and the probation services, the latter when it concerns the return of the prisoner to society. In this regard, United Nations Standard Minimum Rule 49 states (Office of the United Nations High Commissioner for Human Rights, 1957): "So far as possible, the personnel shall include a sufficient number of specialists such as psychiatrists, psychologists, social workers, teachers and trade instructors. The services of social workers, teachers and trade instructors shall be secured on a permanent basis, without thereby excluding part-time or voluntary workers."

In addition to the fundamental provision of forensic health care for all prisoners, forensic psychiatric care is required for those who need it. Examples are mentally ill offenders with an indication for antipsychotic medication or prisoners who are extremely vulnerable during their imprisonment, such as those with learning disabilities or those with offences that may foster victimization by other inmates. These prisoners should be treated according to the state of the art of general psychiatry, which often leads to their transfer to a special ward. As such, many prison systems have wards for drug-dependent prisoners with the aim of preventing the prolongation of drug abuse. Prisoners and staff in such wards should have easy access to a psychologist and psychiatrist. When the mental state of prisoners cannot be prevented from deteriorating further, the transfer to a general psychiatric hospital is required, as forensic ethics demands the prevention of irreparable damage to the health status of detainees due to the imprisonment. This also includes mental health status. This handing over from the prison to a hospital is mostly regulated based on penitentiary regulations.

[13] The United Nations and the Council of Europe have developed regulations for the treatment of prisoners. The United Nations has provided the Standard Minimum Rules for the Treatment of Prisoners (Office of the United Nations High Commissioner for Human Rights, 1957). At the level of the Council of Europe, the main standard-setting document is the European Prison Rules (Committee of Ministers of the Council of Europe, 2006). The European Prison Rules have gone somewhat further than the Standard Minimum Rules by providing more specific guidelines for the treatment of prisoners. Nevertheless, we decided to discuss the Standard Minimum Rules because of the global aim of this chapter.

Specialized psychiatric treatment in prisons may be necessary not only for preventing mental health damage but also for treating mental symptoms that are part of the complex of risk factors. Such forensic psychiatric treatment focuses on the risk factors related to recidivism and, as such, is important for both the prisoner and society. Special forensic hospitals have provided forensic psychiatric treatment for many years, but this is also becoming more common in prisons where treatment programmes are used as a factor in determining the length of stay in prison. However, prisoners cannot be forced to undergo this treatment as they do not represent a danger to themselves or others. That is why the treatment programme should be responsive towards the needs of detainees in a way that it creates motivation.

Achieving a level of care equivalent to that available outside prisons requires establishing outpatient clinics. Not only patients from special hospitals can prolong their treatment there but also prisoners after their release from prison. Even within a certain treatment programme, the possibility of release may arise at an earlier time when compliance with the treatment is good. The visits to these outpatient clinics can start at the beginning on an hourly basis outside prison and then be prolonged to a full stay in the community. In some countries this is called transmuralization or prison programmes. The person stays under the control of the prison service with or without the help of the probation services.

Basic circumstances
The presence of a psychologist, psychiatrist and nurses does not guarantee good mental health. After all, in daily life most people hardly ever see these professionals and are still able to maintain good mental health. The United Nations has formulated Standard Minimum Rules (Office of the United Nations High Commissioner for Human Rights, 1957) for the treatment of prisoners, which provide further safeguards against the deterioration of mental health. The basic principle of the rules is that there shall be no discrimination on the basis of race, colour, sex, language, religion, political or other opinion, national or social origin, property, birth or other status and that, on the other hand, it is necessary to respect the religious beliefs and moral precepts of the group to which a prisoner belongs (Standard Minimum Rule 6). Adherence to this rule is essential for mental health promotion. With general health in mind, it is also essential to adhere to the following rules:

- Prisoners shall be kept in rooms that are sufficiently large and sufficiently lighted, heated and ventilated (Standard Minimum Rule 10).
- Adequate bathing and shower installations shall be provided so that every prisoner may be enabled and required to have a bath or shower [...] at least once a week (Standard Minimum Rule 13).
- Prisoners shall be provided with water and with such toilet articles as are necessary for health and cleanliness (Standard Minimum Rule 15).
- In order that prisoners may maintain a good appearance compatible with their self-respect, facilities shall be provided for the proper care of the hair and beard, and men shall be enabled to shave regularly (Standard Minimum Rule 16).
- Prisoners shall be provided with a separate bed, and with separate and sufficient bedding which shall be clean when issued, kept in good order and changed often enough to ensure its cleanliness (Standard Minimum Rule 19).
- Every prisoner who is not allowed to wear his own clothing shall be provided

with an outfit of clothing suitable for the climate and adequate to keep him in good health. Such clothing shall in no manner be degrading or humiliating (Standard Minimum Rule 17).
- Every prisoner shall be provided at the usual hours with food of nutritional value adequate for health and strength, of wholesome quality and well prepared and served, and drinking-water shall be available to every prisoner whenever he or she needs it (Standard Minimum Rule 20).

Many prisons do not even comply with these minimum rules. However, they are essential standards for basic care and should be the first yardstick to ensure reasonable, fair and humane care in places of compulsory detention.

The Standard Minimum Rules do not fully guard against mental health deterioration and they mean little for mental health promotion. But what does ensure good mental health in prisons? Research on prisoners' needs provides an answer to this question, as research in different types of prison regimes and different countries has revealed quite consistent patterns of needs among prisoners (Toch, 1977).
- The most important thing prisoners need is reliable, tangible assistance from people and settings and services that facilitate self-advancement and self-improvement. Thus, personal development and respect from other people is of the utmost importance for prisoners.
- The next most important need is the need for being loved, appreciated and cared for: a desire for intimate relationships that provide emotional sustenance and empathy.
- The third-ranked need is the need for activity and distraction: the need for maximizing the opportunity to be occupied and to fill time.
- Depending on local circumstances, the need for safety and the need for environmental stability and predictability also may be important.
- Needs for privacy or autonomy are usually less important needs of prisoners.

Some United Nations Standard Minimum Rules are in full accordance with the top three needs of prisoners. With regard to self-advancement and self-improvement, prisoners' most important need, the United Nations states (Office of the United Nations High Commissioner for Human Rights, 1957) that sentenced prisoners must receive treatment that encourages their self-respect and develops their sense of responsibility (Standard Minimum Rule 65). To this end, all appropriate means shall be used, including religious care in the countries where this is possible, education, vocational guidance and training, social casework, employment counselling, physical development and strengthening of moral character, in accordance with the individual needs of each prisoner, taking account of social and criminal history, physical and mental capacities and aptitudes, personal temperament, the length of sentence and prospects after release (Standard Minimum Rule 66). In addition, access to a qualified representative of any religion shall not be refused to any prisoner (Standard Minimum Rule 41).

With regard to prisoners' need for being loved, appreciated and cared for, the United Nations states that prisoners shall be allowed under necessary supervision to communicate with their family and reputable friends at regular intervals, both by correspondence and by receiving visits (Standard Minimum Rule 37).

The following rules address the prisoners' need for activity and distraction:
- Every institution shall have a library for the use of prisoners, adequately stocked with both recreational and instructional books, and prisoners shall be encouraged to make full use of it (Standard Minimum Rule 40).
- Every prisoner who is not employed in outdoor work shall have at least one hour of suitable exercise in the open air daily if the weather permits (Standard Minimum Rule 21-1).
- Young prisoners, and others of suitable age and physique, shall receive physical and recreational training during the period of exercise. To this end space, installations and equipment should be provided (Standard Minimum Rule 21-2).

There is reason to believe that these measures have a major impact on prisoners' mental well-being as they are likely to positively influence the individual's own emotional resilience, which varies from one person to another, and for every individual at different times, depending on external and internal factors. Practical ways of enhancing the individual's emotional resilience therefore include (WHO Regional Office for Europe, 1999):
- access to sports and fitness facilities;
- opportunities to benefit from education and obtain qualifications;
- vocational training and help in obtaining employment after release;
- opportunities to participate in the arts;
- balanced diets;
- access to health care;
- reduced substance abuse or dependence;
- access to drugs and alcohol detoxification and rehabilitation programmes and to opioid maintenance programmes;
- practice in social skills;
- assistance in coping with strong or destructive feelings such as guilt and anger;
- supportive relationships with, and good role models from, staff;
- advice and education on relationships, including parenting;
- opportunities to gain insight into their own offending behaviour;
- opportunities to reflect and take stock of their lives, with support in making changes;
- opportunities to practise the constructive, enjoyable and fulfilling use of time, for example in involvement in the arts or exercise; and
- opportunities for socially useful activity, for example through peer support or community involvement.

Staff training

Many prison systems struggle with the problem of large caseloads and insufficient numbers of mental health professionals (Blaauw et al., 2000). For most prisons, transferring prisoners to specialized institutions is considered to be the best way to deal with potentially problematic prisoners. However, only a few prisoners with mental disorders can be transferred, leaving the vast majority of mentally troubled prisoners to remain in the prisons. Consequently, correctional staff members are made responsible for the daily care of these prisoners. This makes it very important that all correctional staff receive training in dealing with prisoners with mental disorders and in responding to suicidal or aggressive gestures. In this regard, Standard Minimum Rule 47 states:

(1) The personnel shall possess an adequate standard of education and intelligence. (2) Before entering on duty, the personnel shall be given a course of training in their general and specific duties and be required to pass theoretical and practical tests. (3) After entering on duty and during their career, the personnel shall maintain and improve their knowledge and professional capacity by attending courses of in-service training to be organized at suitable intervals.

Especially when there is a shortage of mental health staff, sufficient numbers of correctional staff should be trained to recognize mental abnormality. Using screening instruments is desirable in diagnosing abnormality, certainly in cases in which nurses or specially trained prison officers perform assessments. For instance, the Screening Instrument for Suicide Risk (Blaauw et al., 2001) is an eight-item checklist to assess whether prisoners are at high risk for suicide, and the Jail Screening Assessment Tool (Nicholls et al., 2005) is a semi-structured interview designed to identify mental health problems and risk for suicide, self-harm, violence and victimization among new admissions to pretrial facilities. Prison staff would benefit from receiving training in administering these instruments. In all cases, however, prison personnel should adhere to the principle that transferring prisoners to specialized institutions is better than caring for them in their own facilities.

Prison personnel should receive extensive training in recognizing what imprisonment can cause and in how to collaborate with professionals from other disciplines in prisons. The prison situation has indeed severe disadvantages for the treatment of mentally disordered prisoners due to its being closed off from the world, having non–health care staff and the limited extent to which social workers can be used. The monotony of the daily routine and the activities provided offer prisoners with mental disorders who suffer from psychoses (impaired reality testing, delusions and hallucinations) or personality disorders (deviant behaviour and experiencing with impulsivity, aggression and egocentricity) no opportunity for developing alternative behaviour. The prison environment provides no distraction from what may be a stereotypical way of thinking, feeling and behaving. In particular, the long amounts of time that prisoners spend in their cells can be monotonous, numbing and terrifying. Even if people with mental disorders "sit quietly in their cell" and are therefore not a nuisance to the staff, this does not mean that their disorder is improving or that their disorder will remain constant. It is a semblance of adjustment that leads to the prisoners not being registered as being a "handling problem". After an initial protest, fear of loneliness leads to lack of activity, depression and a pathological tendency to keep to oneself. Detention also has a negative effect on mentally healthy people, but their mental resistance is greater and more flexible. Nevertheless, even they may develop psychosomatic symptoms that should be regarded as adjustment disorders; these disappear once the detention has ended.

If prisoners refuse to accept medication, after participation in the decision and being provided with full information about the proposed treatment, the problem arises as to whether it can be administered against their wishes. A person cannot be forced to undergo treatment unless there are signs of acute danger or the threat of danger for themselves or others. The use of coercion, allowing the person to choose between the two evils of isolation or medication, is then the only possibility for forcing a solution (Moerings, 1994). A broad, multidisciplinary discussion, involving the medical and ethical aspects of the individual case, then becomes necessary. In this aspect, prison staff should be well educated, as staff members are directly concerned with the daily general contacts with and care of the prisoners. Confidence in their own expertise and their capacity to handle urgent situations of increasing violence give them a central role in decision-making for seclusion or more attention and monitoring for a violent person on the ward.

When intervention in the form of compulsory treatment is nevertheless called for, such as with forced medication, then detention in a psychiatric hospital or in a special nursing ward within the prison should be requested. In these cases, specialized control and care should be given in administering medication and applying constraint. Restraint and isolation do not in themselves promote recovery from mental deterioration; they are only useful in that they provide a solution to acute and physical violence by rendering the person concerned physically powerless. Afterwards, structural long-term solutions have to be found as quickly as possible. The most obvious is, if medically indicated, the administration of psychotropic medication. This is particularly the case for psychotic people: disorders involving delusions, mania, agitation or pathological aggression, since medication can usually considerably improve them. The crucial issue here concerns the question as to when the acute danger can be said to have been reduced to such an extent that treatment with antipsychotic medication should be terminated. There is, after all, a considerable risk that when the medication is stopped the mental state will again deteriorate so that a dangerous situation will re-occur, after which treatment will have to be restarted. In these cases continuing the treatment is preferable. Thorough knowledge of the case history regarding previous danger and previous treatment indications is indispensable in such cases.

Conclusion
Reducing mental harm and promoting mental health requires that prison authorities, health authorities and prison staff acknowledge that the preventive treatment and health care provided to prisoners should be equivalent to those provided to the community in general. In prison, different levels of care should be available, sufficient numbers of specialists should be present and the United Nations' Standard Minimum Rules for the Treatment of Prisoners should be adhered to. However, the best safeguard is in place when all prison personnel are carefully selected and adequately trained in mental harm reduction and mental health promotion. Prison personnel form the backbone of mental harm reduction and mental health promotion in prisons

Mental health promotion in prisons: a checklist
The WHO European Health in Prisons Project developed a list of the following ten positive contributions to prisoners' mental health.

1. Reception
Reception into any type of prison can be a traumatic and frightening experience – even if a prisoner has simply been moved from another prison. The reception area and procedures should be organized in such a way as to minimize mental distress.

Wherever possible, facilities should be provided to enable prisoners to make early contact with their families. Experience has indicated that the risk of suicide is particularly high in the first month a prisoner spends in a new prison, with heightened risk during the first days. Reception staff should be trained to detect signs of mental illness and acute distress and to take appropriate action.

Early opportunities should be found to impart information crucial to the maintenance of prisoners' health, on such matters as sexual health and the dangers of sharing syringes and information on what to do and whom to approach if they feel depressed or anxious. Procedures should ensure that all prisoners receive and understand the information given and that, so far as possible, the information is provided in accordance with their cultural traditions. (For example, in some cultures talking freely about sexual matters is not acceptable.)

2. Induction
There should be a well-organized procedure to introduce prisoners to the regime of the prison in such a way as to support and optimize their ability to cope with prison life. Information, for example on sexual health and the dangers of sharing syringes and on what to do if they feel depressed or anxious, which should have been given to prisoners during the reception process, should be reinforced during the induction period. Again, the information should be in a language and cultural setting understandable to the prisoners. Wherever possible, prisoners should be encouraged and helped to make and maintain contact with their families and friends outside prison.

3. A clean environment
The environment of the prison should give a clear message to prisoners that management and staff have positive expectations of them and respect for them. An uncared-for environment lowers self-esteem.

4. A controlled environment
Staff must be in charge of the whole prison at all times. Overcrowding and poor design can contribute to loss of control by staff and bullying and mobbing by inmates, particularly where cell-sharing is unavoidable. Prisons should adopt clear anti-bullying strategies, including support for victims of bullying, and should pay due regard to prisoners' histories (for example, whether a prisoner has a history of violence, especially of an extreme, sexual or irrational kind, or bullying, including emotional bullying) before requiring other prisoners to share their cells. In cases where such a prisoner has to share a cell, staff must ensure the safety of those in their charge by monitoring the situation closely and being available to provide help if needed.

5. Management and staff: support for prisoners
Supporting individual prisoners as they serve their sentences and look towards their eventual release should be an important part of the work of prison officers. Key worker, mentor, supporter and personal officer schemes all require staff to take on this role. Ability in this area should be looked for in potential new recruits. Staff should be trained, supported and given appropriate recognition and reward for this aspect of their work. Time should be built into the regime of the prison for staff

to listen to prisoners and deal with their questions and complaints. Staff members also require training in basic mental health issues and in recognizing and dealing with mental disorder.

Staff should be alert to signs of prisoners undergoing an emotional crisis and in need of extra support – following, for example, disturbing news from their families or an assault in prison – and management should ensure that such support is provided. Someone should be available to talk to such prisoners and help them to cope with the feelings aroused. Prison health care centres may be used to provide short-term accommodation in such circumstances, with staff on hand to help the prisoner. Stress counselling, as well as treatment of physical injuries, should always be offered to prisoners following assaults.

6. Management and colleagues: support for staff
Staff need to feel that their individual worth is recognized. They should feel that their work is valued and appreciated, and their concerns understood, by management: these values should be reflected in how staff interact with their colleagues and with prisoners. Support should be available for staff who have been in stressful situations; for example, staff may need counselling after traumatic incidents such as hostage incidents or the discovery of a suicide. Stress counselling, as well as treatment of physical injuries, should always be offered to staff following assaults. Management should be alert to signs of staff undergoing an emotional crisis and in need of extra support – following, for example, bereavement – and should ensure that such support is provided.

7. Contact with families, friends and the outside community
Family and friendship ties are important sources of support and should be promoted. Although imprisonment requires the imposition of some constraints on visits, letters and telephone calls, the conditions surrounding these means of maintaining contact should be kept as normal as possible. Links between prisons and the outside community (for example, through volunteer visitors representing welfare, educational, religious, vocational or leisure pursuits organizations, or events allowing the public into prisons) should be encouraged and facilitated where possible.

8. Activities
Activities should be available to enable prisoners to make the best use of their time in prison.
- Workplaces and classrooms can offer an environment in which prisoners can be kept busy or diverted enough to achieve a temporary mental "escape" from the pressures of imprisonment.
- Educational and vocational courses and physical education have a major role to play in improving self-esteem and adapting prisoners for release. Research has shown the effectiveness of physical exercise in reducing distress and particularly depression, and access to the arts has been shown to have a major impact on self-esteem and confidence, promoting better relaxation, improved sleep, increased energy and improved anger management.
- Education in parenting skills can help to prevent the perpetuation of cycles of parental abuse and neglect, which can contribute to mental illness and criminal behaviour.
- Training people to forestall depression by such means as cognitive therapies,

coping skills and life skills can significantly improve mental health by promoting self-help.

Religious and spiritual beliefs can contribute significantly to mental well-being. Staff should respect the spiritual beliefs of prisoners, and opportunities and facilities should be provided for practising religion and for developing spiritual awareness.

9. Privacy and confidentiality

Some opportunities should be provided for personal space and privacy. Whenever necessary, (for example during medical consultations), prisoners should be interviewed in private rather than in the presence of other prisoners, and whenever possible in the absence of prison discipline officers. Confidentiality must be seen to be respected.

10. Individuality

Prisons should make choices available to prisoners, to the extent that this is feasible within the constraints imposed by custody. Where staff must handle prisoners' personal property they should do so with due care, respect and sensitivity.

References

Blaauw E, Kerkhof A, Vermunt R (1998). Psychopathology in police custody. *International Journal of Law and Psychiatry*, 21(1):73–87.

Blaauw E, Roesch R, Kerkhof AJFM (2000). Mental health care in European prison systems. *International Journal of Law and Psychiatry*, 23:649–663.

Blaauw E et al. (2001). Identifying suicide risk in penal institutions in the Netherlands. *British Journal of Forensic Practice*, 3(4):22–28.

Committee of Ministers of the Council of Europe (1998). *Recommendation No. R (98) 7 of the Committee of Ministers to Member States concerning the ethical and organisational aspects of health care in prison (adopted by the Committee of Ministers on 8 April 1998)*. Strasbourg, Council of Europe, 1998.

Committee of Ministers of the Council of Europe (2006). *Recommendation No. R (2006) 2 of the Committee of Ministers to Member States on the European Prison Rules (adopted 11 January 2006)*. Strasbourg, Council of Europe.

Fazel S, Danesh J (2002). Serious mental disorder among 23000 prisoners: systematic review of 62 surveys. *Lancet*, 359,545–550.

Ministry of Justice, the Netherlands (2003). *Gezondheidzorgvisie DJI [Health care vision of the Service of Justice Institutions in the Netherlands]*. The Hague, Ministry of Justice.

Moerings M (1994). Isolatie: Noodsprong of beleid? Afzondering in de FOBA [Isolation: necessary or policy? Isolation in the FOBA] In: Koenraadt F, ed. *Psychiatrisch Juridisch Gezelschap, Behandeling of straf? [Psychiatric judicial company, treatment or punishment?]* Arnhem: Gouda Quint:169–176.

Nicholls TL et al. (2005). *Jail Screening Assessment Tool (JSAT): guidelines for mental health screening in jails.* Burnaby, BC, Mental Health, Law, and Policy Institute, Simon Fraser University.

Office of the United Nations High Commissioner for Human Rights (1957). *Standard Minimum Rules for the Treatment of Prisoners. Adopted by the First United Nations Congress on the Prevention of Crime and the Treatment of Offenders, held at Geneva in 1955, and approved by the Economic and Social Council by its resolution 663C (XXIV) of 31 July 1957 and 2076 (LXII) of 13 May 1977.* Geneva, Office of the United Nations High Commissioner for Human Rights (http://www.unhchr.ch/html/menu3/b/h_comp34.htm).

Toch H (1977). *Living in prison: the ecology of survival.* New York: Free Press.

WHO Regional Office for Europe (1999). Mental health promotion in prisons: a consensus statement. In: *Mental health promotion in prisons: report on a WHO meeting, The Hague, the Netherlands, 18–21 November 1998.* Copenhagen, WHO Regional Office for Europe (http://www.euro.who.int/prisons/publications/20050610_1, accessed 15 September 2006).

WHO Regional Office for Europe (2005). *Mental Health Action Plan for Europe. Facing the Challenges, Building Solutions* (http://www.euro.who.int/document/mnh/edoc06.pdf).

24. Dental health in prisons - *Amit Bose and Tony Jenner*

Key points
- Having good dental health is as important for prisoners as it is for the rest of the population
- Prisons should offer a comprehensive dental health care service based on patients clinical needs
- Prisons should provide an appropriate range of dental services
- Prison administrators should be aware of and responsive to the dental health needs of different prison populations
- Prison administrators should continually endeavour to improve dental health services and be aware of indicative growth resources for prison population
- Prisons should work to reduce health inequalities as inequalities do still exist matched to areas of social deprivation
- Prisons should offer open access to information about services and treatments.
- A large percentage of the prison population enter prison with poor oral health
- Untreated disease among prisoners is greater than general population from similar social backgrounds
- Dental attendance among prisoners is less than general population

Introduction

Prisoners have significantly greater oral health needs than the general population. Many prisoners are unemployed before being sentenced and come from communities with a high level of social exclusion. Their high needs and the nature of prison stays lead to high levels of demand for emergency, urgent and routine care. The demand on prison dental services has continued to increase in many countries, especially because the numbers of sentenced offenders have increased and hence the need to be more responsive to their clinical needs.

The commitment of dentists and the dental team is central to the future of dentistry within prison services. Prisoners' dental health needs are comparatively high compared with the population outside prison, and providing appropriate dental services is an essential part of prison health services. Several factors contribute to these needs both before incarceration and during the sentence itself, which are outlined in more detail later in this publication. This chapter offers to help those working with prisoners:
- to improve the quality of dental care in prisons by ensuring that high standards of quality are in place based on clinical quality assurance and robust audit trails;
- to work to raise the awareness of oral health throughout the prison, including among prisoners and prison staff; and
- to recognize dental services as an integral part of comprehensive health services for prisoners.

Dental health needs in prisons

Many prisoners enter prison with poor oral health requiring urgent treatment. This may be due to limited knowledge about good oral health practices. There needs to be a balance in giving priority to emergency and urgent cases over routine care and the length of the sentence. If routine care is neglected, the emergency needs risk continuing to increase.

Alcohol, smoking and substance misuse also contribute to poor oral health. Excessive alcohol consumption, particularly spirits, and tobacco use increase the prevalence and severity of periodontal disease and are by far the greatest risk factors for oral cancer. Substance misuse contributes to high levels of tooth decay and gum disease. Prisoners with substance misuse problems are likely to report toothache very soon after entering prison, as any opiate drugs they took suppressed the toothache.

A dental service provided by a qualified dental team must be available to all prisoners and delivered according to the patients' dental needs and length of sentence. Priorities must be created through a local process of assessing oral health needs.

Challenges in providing dental care to prisoners

Fig. 12.1. Issues and key areas for action in providing dental care to prisoners

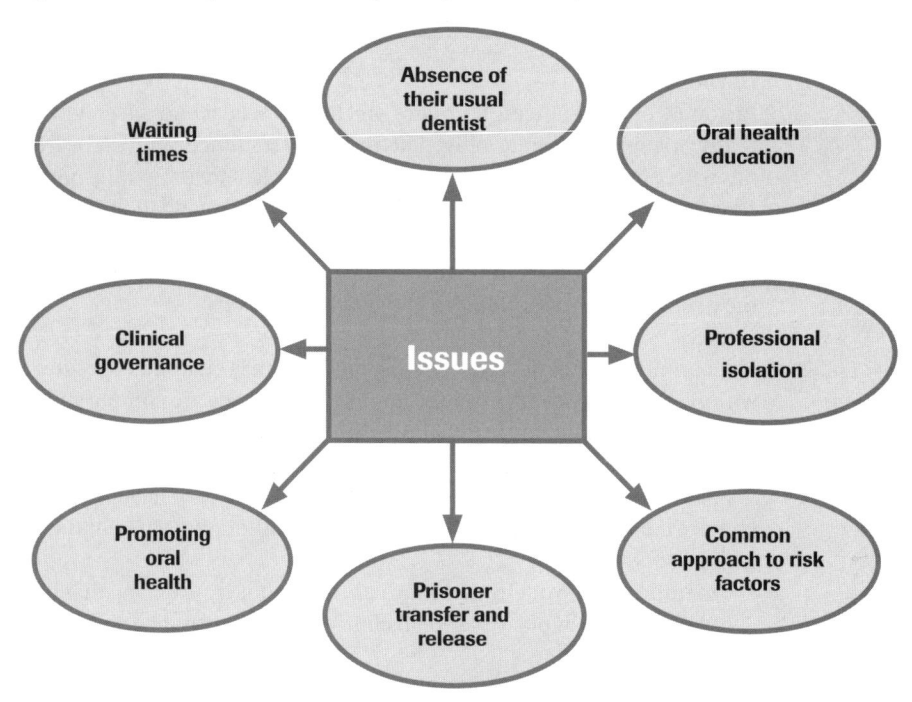

Although dental health has improved considerably in western Europe during the past 30 years, inequality still exists linked to areas of social deprivation. Several factors contribute to prisoners' dental health needs both prior and during the sentence itself. Research has shown that 50% of prisoners are likely to be unemployed before sentencing and enter prison with poor oral health. Further, untreated dental decay is about four times greater in the prison population than the general population from similar social backgrounds. Prior to incarceration, prisoners have lower attendance at dental services than the general population.

The resources to meet dental needs are often stretched, and the ways the services are provided sometimes means that the available resources are not always used efficiently. Prison services therefore face challenges in providing dental services to prisoners (Fig. 12.1).

- Prisoners tend to know their rights and can be very demanding clients and may even take legal action if they feel that they are not being provided with the services to which they are entitled.
- High turnover and growth in the prison population can affect the delivery of dental care for those who need it the most. Prisoners are often unable to reach the top of the waiting list for treatment and are subsequently transferred elsewhere only to be at the bottom of another waiting list. Prisons also have progressively more difficulty in keeping pace with the increased demand for dental care in relation to the increase in the number of inmates.
- Security and factors such as prisoner supervision, security checks on dentists and checks on dental instruments before and after sessions can affect actual patient treatment times. Transporting prisoners to their dental appointments can also be complicated, often resulting in cancellation and non-attendance.
- Resources comprise a major barrier in promoting oral health in prisons. Part of the problem is the length of time prisoners have to wait for treatment, which then leaves practically no time for dentists to promote preventive dentistry.

Oral health promotion

Fig. 12.2. Improving oral health: key areas for action

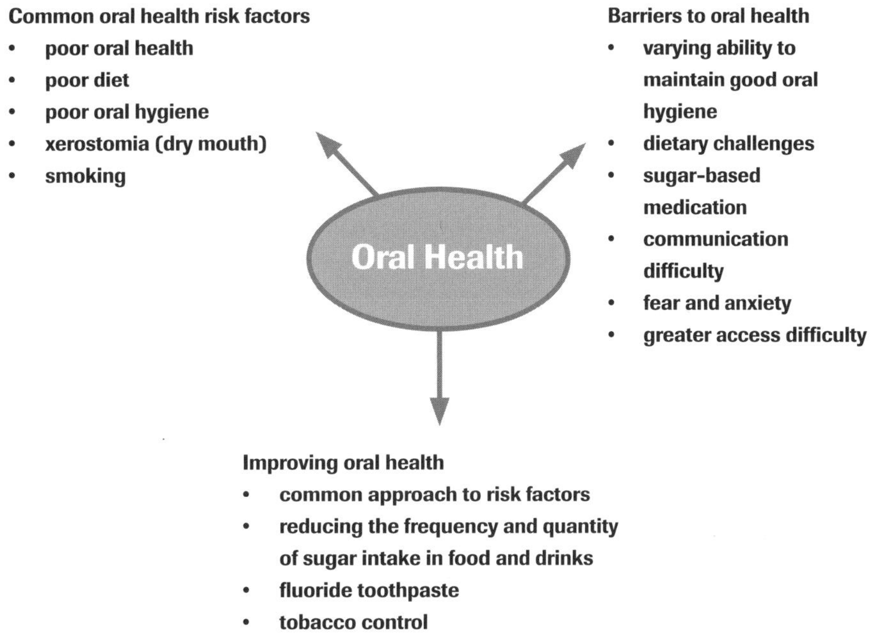

Common oral health risk factors
- poor oral health
- poor diet
- poor oral hygiene
- xerostomia (dry mouth)
- smoking

Barriers to oral health
- varying ability to maintain good oral hygiene
- dietary challenges
- sugar-based medication
- communication difficulty
- fear and anxiety
- greater access difficulty

Oral Health

Improving oral health
- common approach to risk factors
- reducing the frequency and quantity of sugar intake in food and drinks
- fluoride toothpaste
- tobacco control

Many of the main factors that can lead to poor oral health are also common risk factors for other diseases, emphasizing the need to include oral health in initiatives designed to promote health in general.

Low levels of literacy among the prisoners means that many cannot read health care information leaflets that may be given to them unless they are designed for the correct reading age. A strategy to use peers or advocates to promote the health message could be useful.

A range of factors influence what people eat and drink but cost, availability, access and clear information are very important. One particular concern is high levels of sugar consumption, particularly among people living in institutions. Eating a healthy balanced diet containing plenty of fruit and vegetables, low in fat, salt and sugar and based on whole-grain products is important for promoting good general health, including oral health.

Good oral health enables individuals to communicate effectively and is important in overall quality of life, self-esteem and social confidence.

Organization of prison dental services
All prisons should provide support for dentists working within a prison environment by ensuring that there is an effective induction programme. All prisons should ensure that dentists have the appropriate qualifications and work within a clinical quality assurance framework.

All prisoners should receive dental care appropriate to their needs. Prisoners sentenced for a long stay and pregnant and nursing mothers can expect a full range of treatment commensurate with that available within the local regulations.

A different policy can be followed for prisoners on remand or sentenced to six months or less and prisoners within six months of their release. Their treatment planning should take into account the fact that, if treatment is commenced, the work may not be completed before the prisoner moves on.

Prison health care staff should be more involved in oral health promotion (Fig. 12.3).

Fig. 12.3. Good practices in oral health promotion

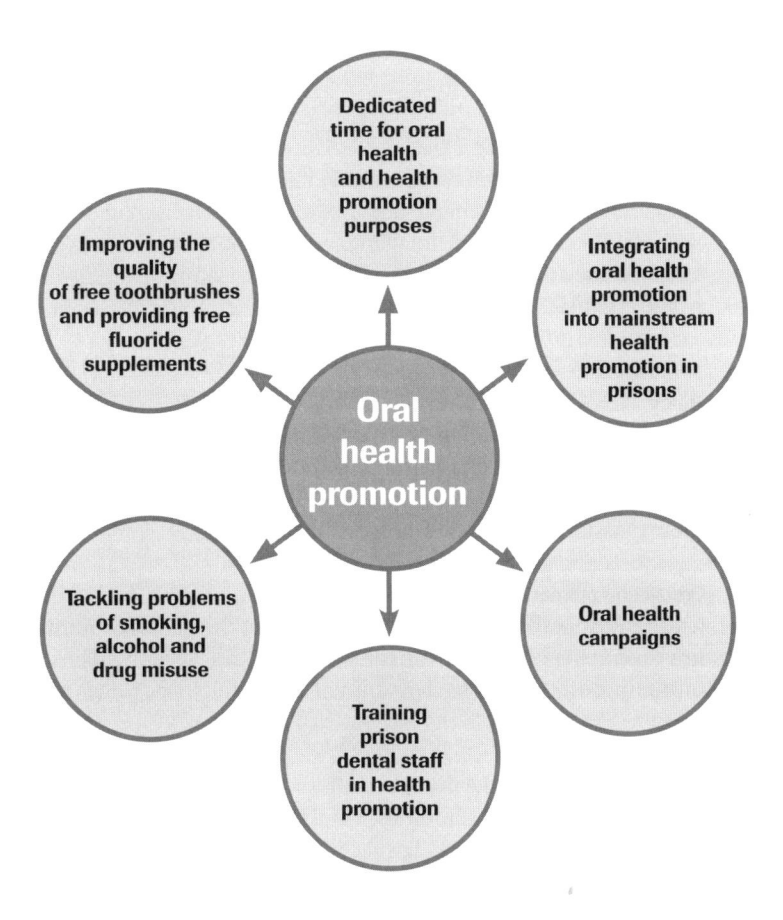

- Dedicated time for oral health and health promotion purposes
- Integrating oral health promotion into mainstream health promotion in prisons
- Oral health campaigns
- Training prison dental staff in health promotion
- Tackling problems of smoking, alcohol and drug misuse
- Improving the quality of free toothbrushes and providing free fluoride supplements

(Central: Oral health promotion)

Models of good practice

This section describes some good practices that have been adopted in prisons (Fig. 12.4). Each prison is different, and what works well in one location may not necessarily work in another.

Induction

On arrival, prisoners get an induction pack and have their general needs assessed to set priorities in dental treatment and inform the dentist of any urgent cases. The information gathered from the prisoners during this induction follows them when they change prison, developing continuity of care.

All new prisoners are offered an examination as part of their induction within Magilligan Prison in Northern Ireland, United Kingdom. All are then offered whatever treatment is required and available under the general dental services. For many of the prisoners, this is an excellent opportunity to reconnect with dentistry, as many of them have been unwilling or unable to access dental care outside. Long-term prisoners are offered a six-monthly review procedure.

Escort
A prison escort service is designed to improve the transfer of prisoners from their cells to the dental surgery. Specialist clinic officers are recruited from the existing pool of security personnel to accompany and assist inmates to the health care facilities. Training is provided, focusing on ensuring that prisoners are searched before and after the appointment and improving the safety of all prisoners while in the health facilities. This helped to improve attendance levels, as prisoners felt more secure while attending their dental appointments.

Triage
Priorities are set among patients using a triage (clinical priority-setting) system. There is no common approach, and systems vary from prison to prison. Well-organized and reliable appointment systems can help to reduce waiting times and to set priorities for treatment according to needs.

Oral health promotion
Oral health campaigns can be integrated into the health promotion and health improvement activities of the prison authorities. Several prisons organize events for promoting oral health, such as annual health fairs, open days and oral health fun days.

In cooperation with the nursing staff, a scale and polish is offered at the end of the smoking cessation programmes. This is a surprisingly successful incentive. The system appears to be working successfully, with relatively few prisoners failing to complete their treatment and the number of emergencies greatly reduced.

Fig. 12.4. Good practices for prison dental health services

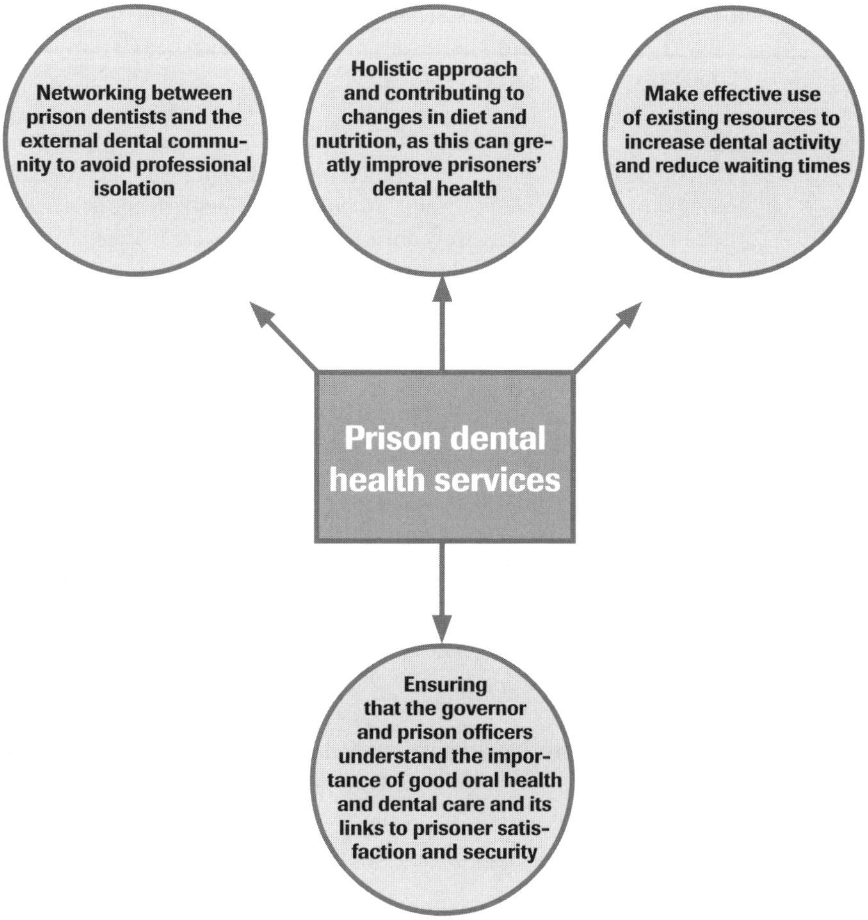

- Networking between prison dentists and the external dental community to avoid professional isolation
- Holistic approach and contributing to changes in diet and nutrition, as this can greatly improve prisoners' dental health
- Make effective use of existing resources to increase dental activity and reduce waiting times
- Ensuring that the governor and prison officers understand the importance of good oral health and dental care and its links to prisoner satisfaction and security

Prison dental health services

Handbook of policies and procedures – Northern Ireland, United Kingdom

A formal written handbook of policies and procedures was developed for prison dental services in Northern Ireland, United Kingdom. The purpose of this handbook is to set out clearly and concisely a set of protocols or policies for many of the day-to-day activities within the dental surgeries in the prison sites in Northern Ireland, United Kingdom. The handbook covers:
- handling requests for routine and emergency dental treatment
- policy on infection control
- handling complaints
- handling and decontamination of laboratory materials
- disposal of clinical waste
- ordering of dental material
- radiation protection.

The handbook acts as an aid to good practice within the prison dental services and is regularly updated to ensure relevance to current clinical practice.

Admission and priority-setting for care – United States of America

The provision of oral health care to prisoners in the United States varies substantially by jurisdiction. Each state has its own unique administration and standard of care. The Federal Bureau of Prisons model was selected, as it represents one of the largest prison systems in the United States.

Admission

Trained health care providers conduct dental screening for all inmates upon arrival. Inmates are interviewed to assess potential oral health needs that are urgent. Inmates responding positively during the interview are referred to a dental health professional for further evaluation.

Within 14 days, each inmate receives an admissions and orientation and examination consisting of a soft tissue, hard tissue and periodontal examination (using the Community Periodontal Index of Treatment Needs). These data serve as a dental and legal baseline of an inmate's oral health at induction. Inmates are also provided information on home care as well as information regarding the access to care at their respective facilities.

Priority-setting for care

With limited resources and a large oral health need, a public health approach to care is essential. Eliminating disease and pain are emphasized. Maintaining existing teeth is a higher priority than the prosthetic replacement of teeth. Patients with less than a one-year sentence are provided palliative care.

Inmates with sentences longer than one year are entitled to routine care. All inmate patients are required to demonstrate good home care before prosthetics are considered or fabricated.

Urgent care

Inmate patients can access urgent care needs on a daily basis. Patients with dental infections, toothaches and trauma can access a health care provider or dentist within 24 hours. During the scheduled work week, inmates can make a sick call appointment to be triaged for dental concerns. Palliative care is provided at these appointments. Urgent care can range from a temporary restoration to extraction. Permanent restorations are placed at routine dental appointments scheduled by the provider.

Routine care

Routine dental care is provided on a fair and equitable basis. Inmates wanting routine dental care submit a request to a staff member and are placed on a treatment list. Inmates are scheduled for treatment planning sessions in the chronological order in which they were placed on the list. After a treatment plan is established, patients are provided dental prophylaxis. Prophylaxis includes sonic and hand scaling, fluoride treatment and comprehensive home care instruction for oral health.

Routine care is conservative. Inmates can receive general restorative care (amalgams and resin restorations), limited endodontics, extraction and removable prosthetics. Aesthetic dentistry, fixed partial dentures, implants and orthodontic dentistry are examples of accessory care. Inmate patients do not normally receive this level of care. Dentists wanting to provide this level of care must submit a request to the Chief Dental Officer of the Federal Bureau of Prisons for review and approval.

Conclusion

The governor, prison officers, health care staff and prison dental team should work together to provide dental care suitable to the needs of the prisoners.

The prisoner's length of stay should be considered when assessing the dental requirements, as this will assist in setting priorities among the dental needs of the prisoners. Oral health is inextricably linked to overall health as well as to self-esteem, and the prison services and dental team are responsible for ensuring that oral health needs are available and accessible as part of the health care delivery systems. If prisoners receive good oral health care, prisoner satisfaction and security will benefit.

Dental services should be recognized as an integral part of a comprehensive health service for prisoners, and administrative support and specific training programmes should be available for dental services as required.

Further reading

Department of Health and HM Prison Service (2003). *Strategy for modernising dental services for prisoners in England.* London, Department of Health (http://www.dh.gov.uk/PublicationsAndStatistics/Publications/PublicationsPolicyAndGuidance/PublicationsPolicyAndGuidanceArticle/fs/en?CONTENT_ID=4005989&chk=nLnjdr, accessed 20 December 2006).
Harvey S et al. (2005). *Reforming prison dental services in England: a guide to good practice.* London, OPM (http://www.opm.co.uk/download.shtml, accessed 20 December 2006).

13. Special health requirements for female prisoners –

Jan Palmer [14]

Key points
- Female prisoners have complex needs, particularly with regard to their physical and mental health.
- Many female prisoners have mental health, substance misuse and self-injury problems. Health care services in prison are needed that take into account the gender-specific issues and problems these women face.
- In England and Wales, United Kingdom, 90% of women prisoners have a diagnosable mental disorder, substance misuse or both.
- Prisons need to ensure continuity of care.
- The rate of both self-harm and self-inflicted deaths is substantially higher in prisons than in the community.
- Staff working in women's prisons should be aware of the particular risks of self-harm among women in custody.
- It is estimated that at least 75% of women arriving in prison have some sort of drug-related problem at the time of arrest.
- Many drug-using women neglect their health while outside prison and have great needs related to health services in prison.
- It is essential that the health care needs of drug-using women be adequately assessed immediately when they arrive in prison.
- It is essential that the specific hygiene needs of women be met from reception with adequate supplies according to individual need.
- The brief periods most women spend in custody present difficulty in adequately addressing their health care needs while in prison and in making follow-up arrangements upon release.
- A comprehensive package of health care needs to be provided for each new reception

---

Introduction

In many European countries the number of female prisoners has risen significantly over the past decade. On average, women represent 4–6% (with some exceptions) of the total prison population. Although the numbers are still relatively small, women have complex needs, particularly with regard to their physical and mental health. Most prison systems have been planned to cater for the large majority of male prisoners, and the specific needs of women can too often be neglected.

Many women serve short sentences, often for non-violent crime. Others are on remand and not yet convicted of any offence. Turnover is high. Health care services need to be able to respond to the needs of a constantly changing prison population. A comprehensive package of health care needs to be provided for each new reception, and this is particularly challenging given the severity of the problems many prisoners have. Trying to make follow-up arrangements for women upon release

[14] I thank Louisa Snow for assistance in writing portions of the chapter. Further guidance and examples of current evidence-based protocols relating to the clinical management of female substance users in prison can be obtained from the author at jan.palmer@dh.gsi.gov.uk.

is often also a challenge. The sudden and unexpected release of women when they appear in court complicates this issue further.

Complex health needs of women include:
- mental health problems
- suicidal behaviour
- substance use problems
- reproductive health.

Mental health problems
The situation of female prisoners in England and Wales, United Kingdom is as follows.
- A total of 90% of women prisoners have a diagnosable mental disorder, substance use or both (Owen, 2004).
- Nine out of ten have at least one of the following: neurosis, psychosis, personality disorder, alcohol abuse and drug dependence.
- A total of 40% of all women in prison received help or treatment for a mental health problem in the 12 months prior to their imprisonment, which is double the rate for men (Singleton et al., 1998).
- More than 66% of women prisoners interviewed for a national survey were assessed as having depression, anxiety or phobias. The comparable figure in the community is 20%.
- About 50% of women prisoners have some form of personality disorder.
- Singleton et al. (2003) found that, among women who were drug-dependent, 83% of remanded women and 75% of sentenced women had two or more mental disorders.

While court diversion schemes aim to keep women with very serious mental health problems out of the prison system, many such women still find themselves in custody. Forensic mental health services are therefore needed to ensure that these prisoners have access to secure hospital accommodation where appropriate.

Some of the women identified above have enduring mental health problems that require the intervention of acute psychiatric services, which should be comparable with those available in the community but take into account the negative effect that prison is likely to have on the mental state of a woman.

Large numbers of women have mental health issues that are quite satisfactorily cared for by the primary health care teams, and prisons need to ensure the development of these services in line with community practice.

Prisons clearly need to develop services to provide for those with a dual diagnosis, once again taking into account the particular needs and issues of a woman detained in prison. This care needs to be continued upon release, where the needs of the individual may change with increased opportunities for the use of drugs and alcohol.

The remainder of this chapter addresses other specific issues related to mental health.

Suicidal behaviour in prisons
The following are important definitions and facts.
- The terms self-harm and self-injury are used interchangeably to describe any act where prisoners deliberately harm themselves, irrespective of method, intent or severity of any injury.
- The term self-inflicted death is used to refer to all apparent suicides in prison.
- The rate of both self-harm and self-inflicted deaths is substantially higher in prisons than in the community.
- Women are 14 times more likely than men to injure themselves while in prison.
- The early period in custody is recognized as being a particularly high-risk time for self-inflicted deaths.
- A substantial proportion of women in prison have experienced some form of abuse.
- Almost half of women in prison on remand (44%) have attempted suicide in their lifetime, compared with 27% of men.
- Women withdrawing from drugs and alcohol can be impulsive, volatile and unpredictable, leading to an elevated risk of sudden acts of self-injury.

Definitional problems are associated with the various terms used to describe the array of behaviour involving the intention of or actual infliction of harm or injury to oneself (O'Connor & Sheehy, 2000). For the current purposes, the terms self-harm and self-injury, which are used interchangeably, are used to describe any act in which prisoners deliberately harm themselves, irrespective of method, intent or severity of any injury. The term self-inflicted death is used to refer to all apparent suicides in prison custody. This term is broader than the definition of suicide as defined by a coroner and includes all deaths in which it is apparent that the individual's actions led to their death, irrespective of intent.

The rate of self-inflicted deaths is substantially higher in prisons than the rate of suicides in the community. According to the Office of National Statistics, the rates of suicide in the United Kingdom during 2003, for instance, were 18 per 100 000 adult men versus 6 per 100 000 adult women. Conversely, the rate of self-inflicted deaths in prisons in England and Wales, United Kingdom (all ages) was 117 per 100 000 adult men versus 316 per 100 000 adult women (Safer Custody Group, HM Prison Service, 2003). These figures demonstrate the disparity between community suicide rates in the United Kingdom and the rate of self-inflicted deaths in prisons in England and Wales, United Kingdom. Possible explanations for this disparity are discussed below, although the definitional differences described above should be kept in mind. Further, the actual number of deaths in prisons is very small (particularly for women), which means that these data must be interpreted with caution.

The rate of self-harm in prisons is also substantially higher than in the community, again, partly because of definitional differences. In 2003, there were 16 214 reported incidents of self-harm in prisons in England and Wales, United Kingdom, which meant that, on average, 7% of the 73 038 prisoners harmed themselves. Women accounted for almost half of the 7407 reported incidents of self-harm, although they accounted for only 6% of the prison population; they were therefore 14 times more likely than men to harm themselves. Women are also far more likely than men to harm themselves repeatedly; a third of men and half of women who harm themselves do so repeatedly.

Most reported incidents of self-harm (57%) involve cutting or scratching and are, therefore, relatively minor (medically speaking). Nevertheless, a substantial proportion of incidents involve self-strangulation (17%) or hanging (8%). Clearly, all such incidents, but particularly those with a higher level of potential lethality (especially hanging or self-strangulation) can put a prisoner's life at risk, even though this may not have been the intended outcome. There were 50 self-inflicted deaths in women's prisons in England, United Kingdom between 2000 and 2004, 41 (82%) of which were by hanging (Louisa Snow, Women's Team, HM Prison Service for England and Wales, personal correspondence, 2005).

The early period in custody is recognized as being a particularly high-risk time for self-inflicted deaths; about half of prisoners who kill themselves were in custody for less than one month at the time of their death (Crighton & Towl, 1997).

It is well established that a substantial proportion of women in prison have experienced some form of abuse. Further, prior sexual abuse is statistically significantly associated with self- harm or attempted suicide among women prisoners. A significantly higher proportion of women (41%) than men (18%) who had attempted suicide or harmed themselves for other reasons reported having been sexually abused (Snow, 2002).

Almost half of women in prison on remand (44%) have attempted suicide in their lifetime versus 27% of men. A quarter (24%) of the women on remand who reported having tried to kill themselves in the 12 months before imprisonment reported that they had been threatened with violence while in prison versus 9% among those who had never attempted suicide.

Prisoners withdrawing from drugs and alcohol can be impulsive, volatile and unpredictable, leading to an elevated risk of sudden acts of self-harm. In addition to this, women in the post-detoxification phase, which can last many weeks or even months, remain at risk, due to the comparative lack of substances, which prior to arrest were very often their way of coping with life. There is also a well-established relationship in the community between substance use and an increased risk of suicide.

In summary, there is clear evidence of increased risk of suicidal behaviour among women in prison. Reducing these risks is not a simple matter, since the reasons for these acts vary from one person to another. Prison directors need to ensure the following.
- Effective health services, as identified elsewhere in this chapter, must be available for all women in prison.
- A suicide prevention coordinator, with in-depth understanding of the risks of suicidal and self-injurious behaviour among women in prison, needs to be posted in each prison.
- Staff working in women's prisons need to be aware of the particular risks of self-harm among women in custody.

HM Prison Service in England and Wales is currently developing guidance for staff on managing and understanding suicidal behaviour among women in prison. The issues addressed in the other sections of this chapter relating to children, mental health, physical health and substance use all contribute to the vulnerability of women in prison. They are described under the relevant headings with their links to the risk of self-harm identified.

Substance use
Data from England and Wales, United Kingdom show the following.
- Women often neglect their health while at liberty due to poverty and or drug dependence, with the result that when they enter prison they make great demands on the health services.
- A total of 60% of all new receptions required clinical management of their withdrawal.
- Women have complex multiple drug use histories at the time of arrest, with a high prevalence of injecting.
- Estimates indicate that at least 75% of women arriving in prison have some sort of drug-related problem at the time of arrest.
- To safely receive these complex women into prison, it is essential that their health care needs be adequately assessed on the first night of arrival.
- Observation and monitoring of withdrawal or intoxication is an essential part of the early part of clinical treatment.
- Prisons should provide dedicated substance use units staffed 24 hours per day by trained health care staff.
- Predicting whether and when a woman in withdrawal is at risk of potentially life-threatening self-harming behaviour may be difficult, and it should therefore be assumed that all women are at risk.
- Clinical regimens should reflect individual need, and if detoxification is indicated in preference to an ongoing opiate substitute prescription, then the rate of withdrawal should reflect the woman's own view of her ability to cope with this.

The author has collected data (Palmer, 2004) showing that 8592 new episodes of clinical detoxification were undertaken for women being admitted to prison in England, United Kingdom in 2004. Although many of these women were withdrawn completely from their substances of dependence, an increasing number were stabilized onto an opiate substitute maintenance regimen. Approximately 20% of women ask to see a doctor or nurse each day, twice the rate of the male prison population.

Clinical data collected from London's Holloway prison between 1998 and 2003 consistently demonstrated that about 60% of all new receptions required clinical management of their withdrawal. These women were typically using 6–9 substances at the time of arrest, including heroin, methadone, dihydrocodeine, cocaine, crack cocaine, cannabis and benzodiazepines (various types). In addition, up to 50% of these women were also drinking alcohol at dependent levels, and 75% were injecting drug users. Women's prisons across England, United Kingdom have observed similarly severe and complex patterns of drug use, although there is some regional variation. There are recent and increasing reports of women misusing buprenorphine (Subutex®) in addition to the drugs already described. An unpublished study of new receptions undertaken at Holloway in 2001 (Palmer, 2001) indicated that, of the 40% of women who did not require clinical detoxification upon arrival, half were using other drugs such as stimulants and cannabis. It is therefore estimated that at least 75% of women arriving in prison have some sort of drug-related problem at the time of arrest. This is in accordance with a study of women entering European prisons (Fowler, 2001), which also found the same percentage of prisoners reporting a history of drug or alcohol abuse prior to arrest.

The following is an example of a "typical" female drug user arriving in prison from England and Wales, United Kingdom:
- age 17–30 years old;
- remanded for 7–10 days;
- charged with theft, failure to appear or surrender;
- using: heroin 1–2 grams, methadone (prescribed and/or illicit use);
- crack cocaine, benzodiazepines (several types – prescribed and/or illicit), cannabis, 6–10 cans of 9% lager beer and cigarettes;
- using drugs for nine years or more;
- injecting drug user – hepatitis C–positive;
- history of psychiatric treatment and/or self-harm;
- medical complications related to lifestyle, such as deep vein thrombosis, abscesses and sexually transmitted infections;
- boyfriend also in prison; and
- children already removed – often with extended family or "in care".

The original charge is often compounded by the woman's inability to comply with the demands made by the courts with regard to attendance or regular reporting. This is often due to their constant need to keep themselves supplied with drugs and the cycle of intoxication and withdrawal. It is not unusual for a woman to have experienced the loss of a child (death) or to have been subject to violence prior to arrest.

To receive these women safely into prison, it is essential that their health care needs be adequately assessed on the first night of arrival. For those who are at risk of withdrawal, this includes commencing prescribing regimens, to treat adequately opiate, alcohol and benzodiazepine withdrawal. Many women require clinical management of all three substances concurrently.

Observation and withdrawal monitoring is an essential part of this early treatment and has two purposes at this stage. Ensuring that symptoms are being brought under control is important, but monitoring for signs of opiate intoxication is equally important, as this is a constant risk when treating women for whom there is little clear, objective evidence of their previous drug use. This risk is increased when benzodiazepines are concurrently prescribed.

Prisons should therefore provide dedicated substance use units staffed 24 hours per day by trained, qualified health care staff, to care for these women. Ideally, these units should (wherever possible) have open health care–type hatches in all the doors (or similar equivalent constant access) to provide "unrestricted observation"

(HM Prison Service for England and Wales, 2000) at all times. These hatches should allow for clinical observations rather than just security observations to take place. For example, in addition to ensuring that the person is still in the room, does her appearance or behaviour give any cause for concern? The hatches also allow staff to hear what is going on in the cells and can be of particular importance at night, when changes to breathing can indicate the development of a serious medical emergency. Staff need to be able to smell the inside of the cell, in case the woman has vomited etc., and finally it is important to be able to touch the woman and to be able to deliver care through these hatches at times when the prison security state does not permit a cell door to be opened in non-urgent situations.

Following a period of stabilization in the first-stage substance use unit, the prison needs to provide a second-stage unit with the same ability to support and observe women as described above, but by this time this care can be undertaken by non–health care prison staff. During this period, staff should focus on the psychosocial aspect of substance use management, as women are then more stable and clear-headed and can benefit from psychological support and interventions in partnership with the clinical regimens. Progress through this stage should be individually determined, and women should not move to a residential location until they are assessed as being able to manage with reduced support and participate in the general prison regime. Clinical management can be continued once a prisoner is moved to the general part of the prison on an outpatient basis.

Having two dedicated substance use units also provides flexibility in accommodating the fluctuating admission rate seen in prisons. There is no such thing as a waiting list; everyone who arrives must be assessed and treated. Having three levels of care available (intensive phase, second-stage and outpatients) always ensures that there are beds in the intensive first-stage unit to receive all new receptions.

In addition to the physical symptoms of withdrawal, prisoners are often present with complex mental problems throughout this period. They are often volatile, agitated and unpredictable and therefore not easy to manage in an environment with strict rules and restrictions. All staff working with these prisoners need to appreciate the effect the withdrawal is having on a prisoner's behaviour and need to be trained and encouraged to defuse potentially volatile situations, avoiding confrontation as far as possible. Another feature of withdrawal is impulsive behaviour, and this appears to put women at increased risk of self-harm during the early period in custody. A feature of self-inflicted deaths during this period has been that staff frequently report that there were no warning signs of intended self-harm before the incident itself. This presents difficulty in predicting when a woman in withdrawal is at risk of potentially life-threatening self-harming behaviour, and it should therefore be assumed that all women are at risk. The level of support and observation to all women during the first four weeks of stabilization and withdrawal should take this risk into account.

Clinical regimens should reflect individual need, and if detoxification is indicated in preference to an ongoing opiate substitute prescription then the rate of withdrawal should reflect the person's own view of her ability to cope with this. Similarly, benzodiazepine reduction regimens may need to be adjusted to avoid increased levels of anxiety.

This risk of self-harm is further increased during this early period in custody by insomnia, which is an unfortunate, but common and persistent feature of withdrawal. Women often cannot sleep well, but making them as comfortable and supported as possible during the night can reduce these risks. Such measures should include:
- open health care hatches (where possible), as already described, with staff available to observe and support women throughout the night;
- providing in-cell television, with unrestricted use of this throughout the night;
- providing additional bedding, as shivering is common in early withdrawal;
- providing additional drinks and food at night, including hot milk drinks such as chocolate at bedtime and throughout the night if a woman is still awake, since women's appetites return strongly as they recover from the initial onset of withdrawal; and
- providing relaxation tapes for use in the cell at night.

Although these should be offered to all women who require clinical intervention for their substance use problems, some of these risks also apply to regular users of stimulant or cannabis users or other prescribed medication.

Stimulant users, whether using these substances alone or in conjunction with opiates etc., provide yet another challenge, with incidents of cardiac arrest and cerebral vascular accidents being reported. Drug abuse is now known to be a common cause of strokes in young adults, and these women therefore need to be monitored upon admission for hypertension and nervous system abnormalities for at least the first 72 hours. Transfer to an outside hospital should be considered if these observations indicate any cardiac or nervous system risk. Agitation and depression are also common among stimulant users, and clinical intervention may be required to treat these conditions, which may be further exacerbated by detention into custody.

Most substance users also smoke cigarettes, and no matter how effectively clinicians treat the other withdrawal symptoms, women will still become distressed, volatile and impulsive if they go into nicotine withdrawal, the severity of which should not be underestimated.

Pregnancy
Of the 8592 women who were admitted for detoxification in England, United Kingdom in 2003, 216 were pregnant (Palmer, 2004). Due to the amenorrhea often caused by their opiate dependence, many of these women did not realize they were pregnant until they were tested upon arrival in prison before starting opiate substitution. This then not only involves the actual safe clinical management of the pregnancy but the need to provide them with the support and opportunity to adjust to the news of being pregnant.

Some women suffer a miscarriage prior to arriving or upon arrival in prison. This is probably due to the interruption in the supply of opiates caused by the period of arrest. Stabilizing pregnancies where there is a recent history of erratic drug use or where drug use has been interrupted is complex, and prisons should ensure they have robust evidence-based protocols for this.

Women may decide not to proceed with their pregnancy upon arrival in prison, especially where they were previously unaware that they were pregnant. Suitable arrangements need to be made for them to receive equivalent treatment options to those that would have been available to them if they were still at liberty. This should include counselling and support as well as the actual termination itself.

For the women who are opiate-dependent, their clinical management prior to the termination should be in keeping with the general clinical regimens used for all pregnant women. This prescribing should continue until after the termination has taken place, in case the mother changes her mind and wishes to continue the pregnancy.

Following termination, women should be allowed time to recover both physically and emotionally, before the clinical management of their substance use is changed. This would normally be a minimum period of four weeks after the procedure has been undertaken, but for some women it may be longer. Opiate substitute maintenance treatment being prescribed to manage the pregnancy safely should then be reviewed and revised according to individual need. Some women may then elect to undergo a slow withdrawal regimen, whereas others may wish to continue a maintenance regimen to address other needs unrelated to the now-terminated pregnancy. Women who commence withdrawal should do so at a speed with which they can cope, and this should be reviewed weekly and revised according to how they are coping. Regimens should be increased or stabilized if the women do not feel that they can proceed with the reduction.

If the woman leaves custody while still receiving an opiate substitution therapy, then the prison clinical substance use team must make arrangements for this treatment to continue upon release. Similarly, if the woman is transferred to another prison, the clinical regimen should be continued without interruption.

Children
Many women in prison have children with whom they were living prior to their arrest and attempt to continue with their role as a carer from within prison. Although regular phone contact and visits can maintain the family links, the frustration and worry of being unable to interact freely with their children may cause great distress and sometimes desperation for the prisoner. This is often exacerbated by the distance from home due to the comparatively small number of women's prisons, which often results in considerable travelling for the families. The distress experienced by these mothers is yet another factor raising the risk of self-harm.

In contrast, some women who have longstanding and severe histories of multiple drug use have become estranged from their children long before arriving in prison. While engaged in a drug-seeking lifestyle they have not attempted to have any contact with their children, but this often changes when they are in a stable and often abstinent state in prison. They feel guilty about their previous lack of contact and both their drug-using and offending lifestyle, which has led to the separation, and they become very focused on wanting to re-establish a relationship with their children. This is often not practical or desirable for the child, and at times formal care proceedings have progressed to a point where any such contact is prohibited. Faced with this inability to re-establish contact, women may become quite desperate, and without the drugs they have previously used as coping mechanisms, they are again at heightened risk of acts of self-harm.

Some women have given birth just prior to arriving in prison but choose not to bring their babies into custody with them or are prevented from doing so by official child-care proceedings or concerns. These women are at particular risk of postnatal depression, which can be both severe and lengthy in duration, and prison health care teams should closely monitor this risk and provide support.

Sexually transmitted infections
Many substance-using women become involved in prostitution before their arrest as a means of funding their drug habit. Other women have engaged in high-risk sexual activity when intoxicated, cannot remember what partners they have had and have not used condoms and therefore run the same risk of disease.

The level of abnormal cervical smear results appears to be higher than normal among this population of women, many of whom have not followed these up. Prison is often a time when they can be encouraged to accept further investigation and treatment.

Bloodborne viruses
Many women in prison have a history of injecting drug use, with the result that they have run a high risk of exposure to hepatitis B and C and HIV. Hepatitis B vaccination programmes should be on offer in all women's prisons, as should testing for hepatitis C and HIV, along with access to local treatment services.

Most women in England, United Kingdom self-report that they cease injecting upon admission to prison, and this would appear to be supported by security information, where needle finds during a period in custody are rare. It is also in keeping with a study (Singleton et al., 2003) finding that just 2% of all prisoners, both male and female, reported injecting. There are, however, commonly complications due to the consequences of injecting drug use prior to arrest, including abscesses, deep vein thrombosis and cellulitis. A further complication is that women may have started treatment for previous deep vein thrombosis or pulmonary embolism but have interrupted their treatment due to their chaotic lifestyle and drug use. These women then present with acute medical emergencies for these conditions, which then require urgent treatment in an outside hospital.

Many women admitted with a history of substance use require interventions for sexual health and bloodborne viruses. Health services in women's prisons need to be resourced to take account of this particularly high demand, especially in a local prison setting.

Violence
Women are often injured upon admission caused, for example, by violent partners

(who may demand that the woman fund his drug habit as well as hers), prostitution clients or pimps and general high-risk situations encountered on the street.

Women who have been victims of violence before arrest may therefore be suffering from low self-esteem, poor coping skills and lack of confidence. Violence contributes significantly to mental health problems, and abusive partners continue to control and threaten some women in prison. Prisons should ensure that there are domestic violence interventions in place (HM Prison Service for England and Wales, 2002).

General health issues
Infestations of head lice and scabies are not unusual among women who have been living rough prior to arrest. These conditions need to be treated upon arrival in prison, together with good general hygiene, to limit the spread to other prisoners.

Many women in prison are of an age where they menstruate. Many opiate users who have experienced a complete absence of their periods from previous opiate use start menstruating again. This is an additional discomfort, with which they have to cope, alongside any symptoms of withdrawal that they experience. Health care teams need to take account of this in clinically managing these women, providing additional symptomatic relief as required.
Sanitary pads and the like, of a type and quantity that the woman finds acceptable, needs to be freely available and easily accessible to women at all times. Some women may have difficulty in approaching male staff to request these items, and prisons need to take account of this to ensure that dignity is maintained. The need to shower more frequently at this time should also be accommodated.

Women who have been using drugs before arrest need considerable dental treatment. As they reduce their level of drug use, they become aware of dental pain, which was previously masked by high doses of opiates. If access to dental treatment is delayed, not only is this distressing for the woman but it also presents an opportunity for women to once again seek analgesia of some strength, which inevitably means an opiate content. This can then once again lead to use of or dependence on these drugs.

Many substance users report a history of asthma, probably due to smoking drugs such as heroin, cocaine and cannabis. Many are also heavy cigarette smokers. The stress to the body of withdrawal often exacerbates this condition, and it is important therefore that women have their inhalers in their possession at all times so that they can treat themselves as required.

Managing epilepsy and withdrawal seizures is complex. Many substance users are admitted with a reported history of epilepsy, and for some this can be traced back to childhood, further confirming the diagnosis. Some have not been following their anticonvulsant treatment regularly prior to admission to prison due to their drug-seeking lifestyle. It is therefore important that this treatment be re-established upon reception into prison, but this can be particularly complicated if the prisoner was dependent on alcohol and/or benzodiazepines before arrest.

Other women claim a history of epilepsy for which anticonvulsant treatment has often been prescribed, with both the community prescriber and the woman believing in this diagnosis. Further investigation may reveal, however, that no formal tests have ever been undertaken, and the seizures can often be traced back to drug or alcohol withdrawal. Because drug use in the community has been both erratic and chaotic, anticonvulsants have been prescribed at times when drug supplies have been minimal or interrupted, and over time this has become part of a steady prescription. When the person is received into prison, often for short periods of time, investigating the true cause of the seizures is difficult, particularly as a reduction in benzodiazepines and or alcohol leaves the person vulnerable to further withdrawal fits. The anticonvulsant treatment is therefore often quite appropriately continued, but this in turn reinforces the incorrect diagnosis of epilepsy.

As part of their history of multiple drug use, many substance users were using alcohol and/or benzodiazepines at dependent levels prior to arrest. These women are at risk of withdrawal fits during the early period of their admission and require clinical prescribing for effectively managing both these withdrawal syndromes to ensure they are safely able to achieve abstinence without the life-threatening risk of seizures. These detoxification regimens should be commenced in an inpatient setting, where there is 24-hour health care provision, as described under the general substance use section. Alcohol withdrawal, particularly in the presence of other drug withdrawal, requires this level of care for a minimum of seven days, but may be needed for longer, particularly when the woman has used both alcohol and benzodiazepines together.

Women who have a genuine diagnosis of epilepsy may have been prescribed a benzodiazepine in conjunction with their anticonvulsant as part of their seizure management. This treatment should be continued in prison in accordance with community advice.

Observation by prison health care staff, over several years, of female substance users who also have epilepsy, indicates that if they were previously using benzodiazepines in the community, then as their reduction regimen progresses, fits emerge that were absent before arrest. It is suggested that this effect can be limited if the benzodiazepine reductions are spaced out to take better account of this, but in some cases continuing this prescribing is necessary in conjunction with the anticonvulsant treatment to stabilize the seizures. It seems likely that, in these cases, the community anticonvulsant treatment has been effective only with the large doses of illicit benzodiazepines being used additionally. Anticonvulsant treatment can be adjusted to try and take account of this, but in reality most women are not in prison long enough for referral to neurological specialists, and ongoing benzodiazepine management as part of managing seizures therefore needs to be considered.

All seizures that occur in prison must be reported to health care staff and the woman examined both during and after each event, as status epilepticus can occur, which is a life-threatening emergency requiring transfer to an outside hospital.

Seizures can re-occur during the prisoner's time in custody due to further illicit use of benzodiazepines. Seizures can also indicate other serious medical conditions, and health care staff need to be vigilant and aware of other possible causes of the sudden onset of fits. Pregnant women who have a seizure should always be transferred to an outside hospital for observation.

As a consequence of their drug-using lifestyle, many women admitted to prison are malnourished. This usually resolves when women stabilize and receive constant nourishing food on a regular basis. Further treatment is not usually indicated unless a normal diet cannot be taken. Women will benefit from additional food and drink supplements at night, as previously described.

References

Dijksman A, Blaauw E (1997). Psychologisch disfunctioneren van gedetineerden [Mental dysfunctioning among prisoners]. *Sancties*, 6:317–327.

Fowler V (2001). *Drug services for youth and women in prison in Europe: the impact of the Marseilles Recommendations*. London.

HM Prison Service for England and Wales (2000). P*rison Service Order 3550 – Clinical Services for Substance Misusers*. London, HM Prison Service for England and Wales (http://www.hmprisonservice.gov.uk/resourcecentre/psispsos/listpsos, accessed 15 September 2006).

HM Prison Service for England and Wales (2002). *Prison Service Order 2700 – Suicide and Self-harm Prevention*. London, HM Prison Service for England and Wales (http://www.hmprisonservice.gov.uk/resourcecentre/psispsos/listpsos, accessed 15 September 2006).

O'Connor R, Sheehy N (2000). *Understanding suicidal behaviour*. Leicester, BPS Books.

Owen S (2004). *A scoping exercise for a health strategy for women in custody in England*. Nottingham, University of Nottingham – School of Nursing. Unpublished.

Palmer J (2001). *Urine test results upon reception*. Unpublished.

Palmer J (2004). *Episodes of clinical detoxification*. London, HM Prison Service Women's Team. Unpublished.

Safer Custody Group, HM Prison Service (2003). *Reported self-harm in HM Prison Service in 2003*. Unpublished.

Singleton N et al. (1998). *Psychiatric morbidity among prisoners in England and Wales*. London, Office for National Statistics.

Singleton N et al. (2003). *Drug-related mortality among newly released offenders*. London, Home Office (Findings 187).

Snow L (2002). *Attempted suicide and self-injury in prisons: an exploration of risk factors and motivations*. Dissertation. Kent, University of Kent.

Further reading

Bukstein OG et al. (1993). Risk factors for completed suicide among adolescents with a lifetime history of substance abuse: a case control study. *Acta Psychiatrica Scandinavia*, 88:403–408.

Crighton D, Towl G (1997). Self-inflicted deaths in prison in England and Wales: an analysis of the data for 1988–1990 and 1994–1995. *Issues in Criminological and Legal Psychology*, 28:12–20.

McEvoy AW, Kitchen ND, Thomas DGT (2000). Intracerebral haemorrhage and drug abuse in young adults. *British Journal of Neurosurgery*, 14:449–454.

Palmer J (2003). *Clinical management and treatment of substance misuse for women in prison.* London, Central and North West London Mental Health NHS Trust Substance Misuse Service.

Palmer J (2003). Detoxification in prison. *Nurse to Nurse*, 3(2).

14. Promoting health and managing stress among prison employees - *Heiner Bögemann*

Key points
- Strategies for promoting health in prison have to include the increasingly complex psychosocial problems of prison employees – burnout, alcohol and drug consumption, internal withdrawal and the inability to come to terms with traumatic experiences in daily work.
- Many penal institutions experience substantial absence due to sick leave and have insufficiently health-conscious employees, employees who cannot carry out all work functions and employees with an upcoming early retirement.
- Health promotion in penal institutions should be seen as a continuous area of personnel development. This requires establishing a connection between work in prisons and the health situation of employees.
- Health promotion should be a steady, comprehensive and interdisciplinary process with focus on the job satisfaction of employees.
- If the individual needs of employees are taken into account and they feel that they can obtain assistance if they need it, they usually feel much better, resulting in declining absence rates and less early retirement.
- Efforts to promote health in prisons can considerably reduce personnel budgets and improve the quality of work with inmates.

Introduction

In recent years the health of employees has played an increasingly important role not only in trade and industry but also in authorities such as the police. Institutions feel more responsible for reducing stress and illness due to work pressure. Key words such as "healthy people in a healthy business" or "efficiency through well-being at work" describe some aims of internal health promotion. But the world of employment in European prisons is still far from these ways of thinking and acting, although in these exceptional workplaces promoting the health of staff members and caring for them would be especially very important to guarantee long-term benefits to society.

In the reality of the prison world, the increasingly complex psychosocial problems of prison staff must be considered. Not only the increasing absence rate due to illness is an indisputable parameter but also such phenomena as burnout, alcohol and drug use, internal withdrawal and the inability to come to terms with traumatic experiences of daily work (post-traumatic stress disorder). These developments often lead either to early retirement or to retirement with physical and mental problems. In Germany, preventive health measurement and health promotion could probably avoid at least one third of early retirements.

The growing stress and expansion of duties in European penal institutions require urgent action. Current problems include overcrowded prisons, intercultural conflicts, often released violently, gang crime within the prisons, language problems, drug use, prisons in bad repair, and frequently insufficient staff with training deficits.

Research on the health of prison employees
The relationships between staff working conditions in a prison and their effects on health has been neither fully made a subject of discussion in criminology nor investigated strongly and comprehensively by the social sciences in Europe. Some studies from Anglo-Saxon or Scandinavian countries focus on single aspects of stress, such as the cause of burnout. The stress and health situation of staff members, including behaviour and relationships, has never been fully discussed.

Neglected research on the health situation of European prison employees has caused problems to be ignored, with resulting negative effects on the imprisonment system. For example, some studies show the following paradox: high discontentment is not caused primarily by stress due to working with inmates but by the organizational conditions and relationships between authorities and staff.

Risk factors and stress among prison employees
So far, all studies on the health situation of prison staff briefly outline various problem areas arising from various types of stress. Nevertheless, stress must not be seen as an isolated problem of a single staff member but as the result of the interaction of different stress factors characterizing this special workplace. Sociologically defined, employees are working in a closed and "total system" with a high degree of reflection on themselves (Goffman, 1961).

The general routine of prisoners' life regulates employees' daily work. This work is characterized by strict hierarchies, depersonalized relationships between staff members and pervasive bureaucracy. Old management structures provoke additional stress. Many places have massive communication breakdown, such as between the authorities and guards in prisons. The local management structures and their behaviour towards staff members are often far removed from modern methods of personnel management. Based on this viewpoint, the following phenomena are often typical of prison staff and therefore of particular interest.

Employees in penal institutions have difficulty in building up an intact and positive role identity. They experience a great discrepancy between their demand for an active role in the rehabilitation process and the reality in prisons, which restrict the role of staff to providing services and guard duties.

Analysis of self and external perception of staff and their role expectations shows considerable discrepancies in the demand for their working role, between "guard" and "helper". The lack of public respect and of social esteem contributes to this negative working role identity with manifest role confusion.

Compared with other social work (care or safekeeping), prison personnel are more often critical about their profession. In particular, the strict regimentation of work by rules is regarded as a stress factor. As the responsibility of the correctional officers is often reduced and restricted to duties of provision and guarding, they feel unchallenged. In addition, a poor working atmosphere (lack of loyalty and cooperativeness) and inadequate organizational structures adversely affect job satisfaction and can initiate stress. Satisfaction increases as soon as staff members obtain both more rights to speak out and autonomy and influence on official work and care tasks.

Disturbance in daily communication, especially between different hierarchical levels, initiates stress among many staff members. Communication breakdown must therefore be regarded as a frequent stress factor in prisons. Professional support of staff, such as by supervision measures, encourages the competence of communication and, through this, communication itself. In addition, this support may reduce anxiety and be useful in contacts with difficult inmates and reduce confusion with the professional role and in supporting relationships with strict hierarchical structures. Overall, the social support for employees is inadequate.
The concentration and the interaction of different stress factors in prisons bring about increasing burnout signs among staff, such as reduced ability and depersonalization. All helping professions recognize burnout as a problem, but prison staff especially have an increased risk of burnout. Compared with other psychosocial job profiles, this kind of helping work imposes extreme tension between help and control.

An important factor for the development of a burnout syndrome is the fact that work with inmates often results in failures. Worthy of mention here are more and more complicated clients with an increasing readiness to resort to violence who also bring mental problems into the prison. There are language problems, and in many places overcrowded prisons that provoke additional stress. Staff shortages cause imprisonment to develop more and more into a safekeeping institution that is less successful with rehabilitation measures (guiding principles: clean, safe and full).

Further, there are negative factors, such as low influence and a lack of participation in decision-making processes, inappropriate salary and the feeling of not being challenged by the work. But in the end, the stress caused by institutional deficits, "administrative practices", is more serious than the stress due to contact with prisoners.

Frequent psychosocial risk factors in prisons
Latent stress arising from various factors is very often noticeable in prisons. Continuous stress affects people mentally, physically and cognitively, with results ranging from psycho vegetative exhaustion to burnout. Post-traumatic stress disorder may accelerate this development, especially when the prison climate is characterized by disturbed communication, depreciation of work by superiors, low social team spirit among working groups, lack of corporate identity and organizational parameters, such as overtime accumulating as a result of a poorly organized work process.

On ordinary weekdays in a prison, employees often increase their use of coffee, cigarettes, alcohol and also medication. Sometimes further risk factors crop up such as unbalanced nutrition (fast-food in shift work) and insufficient physical exercise.

Many penal institutions have a latently high level of sick leave, insufficiently health-conscious staff, staff that cannot carry out all work functions and staff with upcoming early retirement. Many staff members have the further problem of thinking they have reached a dead end with poor career prospects with a lack of future training and promotion. In practice, this could be important if fewer and fewer qualified employees are willing to work in prisons.

Promoting and developing employees with health in mind
With complex problems in the background, European penal institutions should see health promotion as a continuous area of personnel development. This requires establishing a connection between work in prisons and the health situation of staff. The aims should be to give employees a feeling of recognition, to support them in attaining results and in a challenging job that must not become an end in itself but actively contributes to the safety of their society.

Health promotion should be a steady, comprehensive and interdisciplinary process focusing on job satisfaction. Through close contact between staff members and inmates, the climate of penal institutions directly depends on job satisfaction, especially among correctional officers. Job satisfaction certainly affects their behaviour regarding inmates. Staff can develop care and counselling programmes (such as social training) for prisoners and support them with more interest and commitment. That would be welcome not only for improving the functioning of the social community but also for economic and administrative reasons as society has to bear the health care costs of prison staff. One day of sickness costs about €200–400 and occupational incidents cost up to €800 daily.

Practical approaches to health promotion: best practices
The following section describes various practical approaches to health promotion in prisons. They document experience from a pilot project carried out in Germany with an analysis of a health centre for imprisonment. The health centre is responsible for 35 penal institutions with about 4000 female and male correctional officers. It is the first health centre of its kind in Germany and works interdisciplinarily.

14.1 The apple as a symbol of health promotion in prisons in Germany

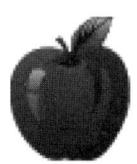

The apple is the logo of the health centre. It stands for personal responsibility in health promotion as well as for disease prevention and prophylaxis. Since "an apple a day keeps the doctor away", the apple is the visual symbol for health care in the penal institution. It also emphasizes preventing illness instead of merely curing it. This fruit has a positive connotation for most staff members.

The focus lies on the practical relevance of small and large steps that can be implemented in prisons independently of size and safety alignment. The measures documented here have been tested over several years in different prisons in Germany.

The priorities of this approach are self-help and the internal use of existing (salutogenetic) resources and the use of non-professionals who are activated within a network. The principle of this practical network job is: "Health promotion in my prison – from idea to action".

This practical approach enabled staff in different hierarchies to be integrated in a self-help system and to motivate personnel in developing and implementing health promotion projects typical for prisons. This participatory activity is interdisciplinary and uses the already available resources for health promotion in prisons and is oriented towards existing job security and regulations governing occupational safety. It is comprehensive community action for health.

So far the "healthy prison" approach has been developed based not only on the Ottawa Charter for Health Promotion (WHO, 1986), which integrates the developments of new public health research, but also on many salutogenetic aspects and resources (Antonovsky, 1988). This enables the professionals of the health centre to react adequately and with flexibility to the complex work risks of prison staff.

Comprehensive health promotion for prison employees

Integrating wide-reaching health promotion measures in the structure of penal institutions requires that all the responsible politicians and ministries support this approach. They should not only realize the meaning and practical use of health promotion strategies but also actively support the implementation of such measures (top down).

At the institutional level, different concepts can be created to develop health management structures. Ideally, all approaches and action strands are interlocked so that a comprehensive health-promoting strategy can be seen in the end as having a lasting effect both on behaviour level (staff) and on relationships (institution). Health management should always be understood as a continuous process aiming at actively integrating as many staff as possible.

Example of a health in prison project with important milestones

Box 14.1 presents in chronological order a development process of health promotion structures in a closed prison in Germany with 400 staff members and 700 inmates from 1996 to 2001.

Box 14.1. Development of health promotion structures at a closed prison in Germany

A study group on health comprising a health research associate, social worker, educator, personnel committee and the administration prepared an informal, interdisciplinary project. The project started with a pilot institution. The logo was chosen as an apple.

The study group visited all departments for several days and intensively analysed working conditions. An information network was set up (non-fiction books, information brochures on such topics as health insurance schemes, the Internet etc.).

The study group was constituted with the institution director, administration, supervisors, the personnel committee, a women's representative, an action group on health promotion, a pastor and the resident physician. Psychosocial care was started, including crisis management, addictive problems and psychosocial care.

All staff members were interviewed by questionnaire. The response rate was 70%. The responses were analysed. A national action group on post-traumatic stress disorder was created. The interview results were presented and discussed with all staff in each prison and department.

The communication infrastructure was improved, including vocational training, training, executive personnel training, preventing dependence, executive personnel training and conferences (on work in the future, communication and other topics).

The psychosocial consultation structures were improved. A back-school was started to encourage back exercises and stress management. Quality and health circles were introduced in each prison.

Staff members were asked about post-traumatic stress disorder and the concept of improving crisis intervention for each prison and in each of the Länder.

Cooperation was begun with WHO and the European Health in Prisons Project, including attending a WHO Regional Office for Europe (1999) meeting on mental health promotion in prisons in The Hague in 1998.

A project report was prepared for the Ministry of Justice. Due to its great success, the project was extended.

Further training outside the prison has been intensified (stress management, health promotion, team efforts, sessions 2–5 days, up to 20 people each). A working group has been created on personnel for better coordination of disease-preventive health efforts, dependence prevention and further training.

The project has been modified in agreement with the Board of Justice. The project content is being extended to two further prisons with about 500 staff members. The size of the target group is now about 900 people.

Help offers for special stress diseases (post-traumatic stress disorder) have been expanded to further institutions. A national programme for crisis intervention is being developed.

Essentials for active health management in prisons

Since 1997, when the first health promotion project started in a prison in Germany, practical experience has shown that different topics should be integrated to form a whole in developing health promotion structures. The most important pillars and practice components proven up to now are mentioned briefly in this section.

Health promotion includes managing stress, preventing illness, integrating occupational safety and health measures and developing them further, consultation with health professionals, comprehensive health care (such as setting up of information networks and libraries in prisons) and further training.

Crisis intervention includes crisis consultation and crisis care (such as after the suicide of a prisoner), founding self-help networks (contacting colleagues after special incidents, such as violence against staff), managing conflicts and preventing crises, ranging from specific training and prevention to intervening in specific crises. A national team for crisis intervention acts and cares immediately for staff in prison whenever required after incidents.

Organizational aspects include communication consultation, team advice, advisory systems of colleagues and non-professionals, interaction training, quality and health circles and organizing supervision, coaching and mediation.

Rehabilitation includes cooperating with representatives of people with disabilities and problems concerning the rights of these people, psychosocial consultation (such as for cancer), preventing dependence and arranging therapy (especially for alcohol use), cooperating with hospitals and rehabilitation centres and helping people to reintegrate into the work process (moving to another workplace and testing working capacity).

Advice on project methods includes initiating internal health promotion projects in prisons, questioning personnel and interviewing experts as the basis of health promotion efforts, preparing regular health reports on physical condition and the state of health promotion measures in each prison, ranking health among some prisons and implementing evaluation and empirical research on the efficacy of the measures developed. Interdisciplinary research cooperation between prisons is being initiated in close contact with universities, advanced technical colleagues and national and international institutions such as the WHO European Health in Prisons Project to improve health promotion measures continuously and throughout Europe.

Health promotion self-help networks in prisons
A central idea is to set up a self-help network in prisons with honorary prison staff for holistic health promotion. The network consists of staff from all hierarchical levels, participating together in an interdisciplinary fashion and based on project management structures. They use:
- non-professionals in consultation and care;
- organizational resources, abilities and interests; and
- internal resources in prison such as previous professional experience and special knowledge of staff from former professions (such as masseur, physician's assistant, nurse, pedicurist and dietitian).

The internal use of existing resources of personnel (staff, specialized social services, doctors, administration, etc.) is important for this idea to let staff first analyse the problems and then develop solutions (Box 14.2). Afterwards, the concerted strategies must be put into action each working day. Staff are thus affected by a problem (passive) and at the same time supported by specialists in solving problems (active). Here the operating principle of quality and health circles is applied and is an important element of health activities in prisons.

> **Box 14.2. Checklist for self-help actions and initiatives in prisons**
> - setting up a health promotion group (quality circle);
> - conducting internal public relations work in penal institutions;
> - setting up health information centres;
> - providing assistance in health target and service agreements;
> - initiating service agreements concerning drug abuse;
> - raising money for work;
> - preparing and implementing an interview of the personnel about their health status;
> - preparing and implementing health days;
> - preparing and implementing information days on such topics as drugs, bullying and stress;
> - preparing stress management seminars;
> - organizing nutrition consultation;
> - organizing fitness and sports;
> - organizing fitness offers;
> - organizing supervision offers for team consultation;
> - promoting get-together activities (such as team parties or hiking);
> - improving nutrition during work, such as fruit in the canteen and a water cooler;
> - encouraging problem and crisis consultation by colleagues;
> - mediating drugs, crisis or debt consultation;
> - setting up regional working groups for exchanging experience;
> - setting up help structures after special incidents and stress diseases (contact to colleagues, debriefing); and
> - conducting non-smoking training.

Continuing education

The activities mentioned above take place not only on site in prisons but are also part of a nationwide continuing education programme. This supraregional, often interdisciplinary further training will increasingly enhance and establish the idea of health promotion. Thematic examples of continuing education being conducted by health centres include:

- health promotion in my prison – from idea to action
- creating and maintaining healthy work and living spaces
- basics of communication
- contact with colleagues as an effective basis of case and service meetings
- personal health promotion and approaches to a healthy life
- coping with death and suicide at the workplace
- people with disabilities at the prison workplace
- supervision – a contribution to improving the quality of professional work
- communication in penal institutions – contact and consultation with colleagues
- health behaviour among men
- mobbing in the working world and in prison
- women in prison jobs (gender mainstreaming)
- traumatic professional incidents and how to cope with them
- stress without end…? Stress management in prison
- continuing education meeting for crisis intervention teams
- from smoker to non-smoker – non-smoking training in 10 steps
- occupational health and safety in correctional facilities.

Results and prospects

Future practical experience with health promotion measures will certainly again prove that only healthy and content personnel provide active assistance in rehabilitation. So far, employees in prisons represent a model for the inmates. The goal of prison sentencing to enable former prisoners to lead a future life in social responsibility without crime assumes that healthy and motivated personnel care increasingly for the health of inmates to enhance opportunities for rehabilitation. This can only be achieved when prison employees themselves are in good physical and mental health and appreciate work done well and corresponding further professional training and development prospects to accompany working life behind the walls.

Considering the individual needs of employees and the possibility of obtaining assistance will ensure that employees feel much better and will increasingly identify with the job content. This will result in declining absenteeism and less early retirement. This will enable considerable savings in personnel budgets, and the quality of work with inmates will also improve.

Ideally, at the national and European level, health promotion projects will be developed that continuously exchange information and experiences and closely cooperate with a growing network across national borders. So far, the WHO European Health in Prisons Project presents an ideal platform for all European countries to strive together towards reaching this target in the future.

References
Antonovsky A (1988). *Unraveling the mystery of health.* San Francisco, Jossey-Bass.
Goffman E (1961). *Asylums. Essays on the social situation of mental patients and other inmates.* Harmondsworth, Penguin.
WHO (1986). *Ottawa Charter for Health Promotion.* Geneva, World Health Organization (http://www.who.int/healthpromotion/conferences/previous/ottawa/en/index.html, accessed 15 September 2006).
WHO Regional Office for Europe (1999). Mental health promotion in prisons: a consensus statement. In: *Mental health promotion in prisons: report on a WHO meeting, The Hague, the Netherlands, 18–21 November 1998.* Copenhagen, WHO Regional Office for Europe (http://www.euro.who.int/prisons/publications/20050610_1, accessed 15 September 2006).